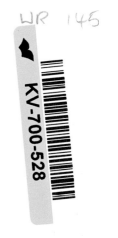

Modern Management of
Common Skin Diseases

This book is dedicated to Ian Sneddon who first fired my interest in dermatology and has influenced many of the authors in this book.

C.F.H.V.

Modern Management of Common Skin Diseases

Edited by

Christopher F. H. Vickers MD FRCP

Professor of Dermatology,
University of Liverpool and
Consultant Dermatologist,
Royal Liverpool and Alder Hey Children's Hospitals,
Liverpool, UK

CHURCHILL LIVINGSTONE
EDINBURGH LONDON MELBOURNE AND NEW YORK 1986

CHURCHILL LIVINGSTONE
Medical Division of Longman Group UK Limited

Distributed in the United States of America by
Churchill Livingstone Inc., 1560 Broadway, New York,
N.Y. 10036, and by associated companies, branches
and representatives throughout the world.

First published 1986

ISBN 0 443 03316 1

British Library Cataloguing in Publication Data
Modern management of common skin diseases.
   1. Skin Diseases
   I. Vickers, C. F. H.
   616.6   RL71

Library of Congress Cataloging in Publication Data
Modern management of common skin diseases.
   Includes index.
   1. Skin--Diseases--Treatment.   I. Vickers, C. F. H.
[DNLM: 1. Skin Diseases--therapy.   WR 650 M689]
RL71.M63   1986   616.5   85–25967

Made and printed in Great Britain by
Hazell Watson & Viney Limited,
Member of the BPCC Group,
Aylesbury, Bucks

Preface

This book is addressed mainly to primary care physicians and is intended as a guide to common dermatoses and their up-to-date management. As the approach has been an international one, a disease may seem rare in one part of the world whilst prevalent elsewhere. It is hoped that all the common dermatoses have been covered.

The main emphasis is on therapy as the title implies. A modicum of clinical diagnostic material has been included, together with the illustrations, to try to help with a difficult diagnosis.

There are several ways of using this book. If the diagnosis is known, it will appear as a chapter heading or in the index. Some chapters are concerned with anatomical sites or geographical areas and these may lead into the appropriate part of the book. Two chapters overview topical and systemic treatments and these deal with specific drugs and dosage regimens. A brief formulary is also included.

I would like to thank all my collaborators for their contributions and for accepting the editing that was sometimes required. I trust this will make for easier reading.

Liverpool, 1986   C. F. H. V.

Contributors

Susan M. Burge BSc BM MRCP
Senior Registrar in Dermatology,
The Slade Hospital,
Headington, Oxford, UK

Ronald E. Church, MA MD FRCP
Consultant Dermatologist and
Lecturer in Dermatology,
University of Sheffield,
Sheffield, UK

John A. Cotterill BSc MD FRCP
Consultant Dermatologist,
The General Infirmary,
Leeds, UK

Rodney P. R. Dawber MA MB FRCP
Consultant Dermatologist,
The Slade Hospital,
Headington, Oxford, UK

Paul A. Dufton MB MRCP
Consultant Dermatologist,
Arrowe Park and Clatterbridge Hospitals,
Wirral,
Merseyside, UK

Susan Evans MD
Consultant Dermatologist,
Newsham General, Whiston and St Helen's Hospitals,
Merseyside, UK

William Frain-Bell MD FRCP
Senior Lecturer in Dermatology,
The University, Dundee and
Consultant Dermatologist,
Ninewells Hospital, Dundee,
UK

Lionel Fry BSc MD FRCP
Consultant Dermatologist,
St Mary's Hospital,
London, UK

Patrick Hall-Smith MD FRCP
Consultant Dermatologist,
Royal Sussex County Hospital,
Brighton, UK

Robert C. Holmes MB MRCP
Consultant Dermatologist,
Coventry & Warwickshire Hospital,
Coventry, UK

Vibeke Kassis MD PhD
Consultant Dermatologist,
University Hospital,
Copenhagen, Denmark

Robert A. Marsden MB MRCP
Consultant Dermatologist,
St George's Hospital,
London, UK

John H. S. Pettit MD FRCP
Consultant Dermatologist,
Kuala Lumpur,
Malaysia

Alan R. Shalita MD
Professor of Dermatology,
State University of New York,
Brooklyn,
New York, USA

J-H. Saurat MD
Professor and Chairman,
Clinique de Dermatologie,
Hospital Cantonal,
University of Geneva,
Geneva, Switzerland

Thomas W. Stewart MB FRCP
Consultant Dermatologist,
Royal Liverpool Hospital and
Lecturer in Dermatology
University of Liverpool,
Liverpool, UK

David Taplin
Professor of Dermatology and
Cutaneous Surgery and
Professor of Epidemiology and Public Health,
University of Miami School of Medicine
Miami, Florida, USA

William R. Tyldesley FDS RCS DDS
Reader in Oral Medicine,
University of Liverpool,
Liverpool, UK

Julian L. Verbov JP MD FRCP FIBiol
Consultant Dermatologist,
Royal Liverpool Hospital and
Lecturer in Dermatology,
University of Liverpool,
Liverpool, UK

Christopher F. H. Vickers MD FRCP
Professor of Dermatology,
University of Liverpool and
Consultant Dermatologist,
Royal Liverpool and Alder Hey Children's Hospitals,
Liverpool, UK

Robert P. Warin MD FRCP
Consultant Dermatologist and
Lecturer in Dermatology,
University of Bristol,
Bristol, UK

Contents

     J. H. S. Pettit

15. **The photodermatoses** 136
     W. Frain-Bell

16. **Psychogenic dermatoses** 157
     J. A. Cotterill

17. **Pregnancy dermatoses** 164
     R. C. Holmes

18. **Bullous dermatoses** 171
     R. A. Marsden

19. **Dermatoses with oral involvement** 180
     W. R. Tyldesley

20. **Dermatoses involving the hair and nails** 187
     S. Burge and R. P. R. Dawber

21. **Topical therapy—a review** 203
     L. Fry

22. **Systemic therapy—a review** 211
     J. L. Verbov

     Formulary 216

     Index 221

D. Taplin

1. Cutaneous Infections

STREPTOCOCCAL INFECTIONS

Streptococcal pyoderma

Clinical features Beta haemolytic *Streptococcus pyogenes*, usually of Lancefield Group A, is the commonest cause of skin infections worldwide. Prevalence is higher in children than adults, in tropical climates and in conditions of poor hygiene. The initiating factor is minor skin trauma. The distribution and appearance of the lesions are dependent on the sites and types of minor injury.

In the tropics insect bites frequently become infected and most lesions occur on the lower limbs (Fig. 1.1). Multiple streptococcal pyodermas of

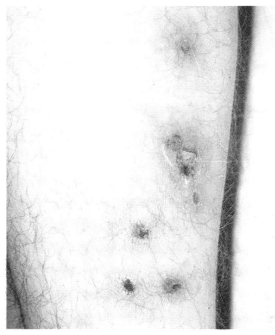

Fig. 1.1 Streptococcal infection of insect bites.

the scalp are associated with head louse infestations and those in scabies are found in sites such as the genitalia, wrists and intergluteal cleft. Knees and elbows are common sites of infected abrasions. Physicians and health care personnel should consider the role of such initiating factors which may require additional therapy or preventative measures.

The initial lesion of streptococcal pyoderma is a pustule, surrounded by spreading erythema. By the time most patients seek medical attention, lesions are purulent, crusted and painful. Removal of crusts reveals a shallow ulcer extending into the dermis. Regional lymphadenopathy is common. Once the lesion develops a crust, it rapidly becomes a haven for pathogenic *Staphylococcus aureus*.

Management

Antibiotic therapy alone for infected scabies, pediculosis capitis or insect bites provides temporary relief from acute infections, but recurrence is the rule if the underlying conditions or environmental insult is not corrected at the same time.

Until the late 1970s it was generally considered sufficient to treat streptococcal pyoderma with penicillins, such as oral penicillin V or long acting injectable benzathine penicillin G, regardless of the concomitant presence of *Staph. aureus*. More recently there is reason to question this approach as many isolates of *Staph. aureus* are now resistant to penicillin. Many cases treated with oral penicillin V now fail to respond to therapy. In contrast, the skin infections in patients treated with cloxacillin heal rapidly.

Geographic variations in clinical response may vary, depending on the frequency, virulence and antibiotic sensitivity of local *Staph. aureus* strains. The emergence of multiple drug resistant strains of *Staph. aureus* in hospitals is well known and is strongly influenced by the types and amount of antibiotics administered in the particular hospital. Similar effects can occur in open communities. It is, therefore, important to monitor clinical response to therapy, and institute periodic antibiotic sensitivity surveys of skin pathogens.

Erythromycin is an acceptable alternative to penicillin but gastrointestinal disturbances may limit its usefulness. Cephalexin is valuable and is well-tolerated in mixed staphylococcal/streptococcal infections. Dicloxacillin may be used with equal efficacy to cloxacillin but the bitter taste of the suspension is not acceptable to many children.

Topical antibiotics or mixtures of antibiotics are of limited value in the treatment of streptococcal pyodermas. They may be useful in preventing infections of superficial abrasions and, theoretically, should reduce the chances of bacterial transfer to other sites of skin trauma or to other persons.

Care of lesions consists of gentle cleansing with soap and water, skin cleansers, or 3% hydrogen peroxide solution to remove crusts, followed by a light dressing to keep the area clean. In the tropics, where wound-feeding flies and gnats play a role in transmission, a coating of silver sulphadiazine cream may be used as an additional barrier prior to application of the dressing.

Streptococcal cellulitis

Clinical features

This is an acute, painful, red, hot, tense swelling of the subcutaneous tissues, usually involving the extremities (Fig. 1.2). The border between affected areas and normal skin is ill-defined. It may follow a localized streptococcal pyoderma, trauma or result from a puncture wound, laceration or friction blister at a distal site. It is usually unilateral. Occasionally, the portal of entry cannot be determined.

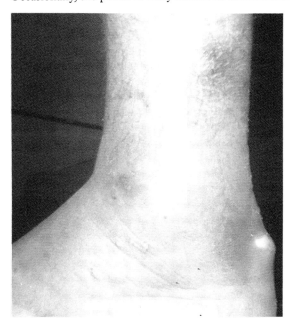

Fig. 1.2   Acute streptococcal cellulitis secondary to infected friction blister.

Management

Streptococcal cellulitis of the lower leg should be considered a medical emergency requiring bed rest, elevation of the limb and high doses of appropriate anti-streptococcal antibiotics, including intravenous administration in severe cases. Circulation may be impaired and rapid treatment is required to prevent permanent lymphatic damage. Lymphadenitis and lymphadenopathy are common. Systemic signs may be minimal but high fever, rigors and other signs may be present.

Erysipelas

Clinical features

This is a more superficial type of streptococcal cellulitis with rapidly spreading erythema and a well-defined border which may have a vesicular element. The involved skin is uniformly hot, bright red, oedematous and painful. In elderly patients, petechiae may be present.

   Erysipelas may occur in the abdominal wall in infants, and the face and limbs are common sites in older children. The lower limb is reported to be involved in half of the adult cases but there may be some confusion with acute streptococcal cellulitis.

The classic form of erysipelas affects the face. Lesions often begin on the cheek and spread across the face to form a butterfly configuration in a few days. At this point, patients usually exhibit signs of toxicity, including high fever, chills, malaise, headache, nausea and back pain. The leukocyte count usually exceeds $15\,000/mm^3$.

Management   Penicillin remains the drug of choice. Mild or early cases may be treated with oral penicillin V, cloxacillin or dicloxacillin. Infants, adults with generalized symptoms and cases involving limbs, where circulation is impaired, may require intravenous therapy. In cases of penicillin allergy, oral erythromycin may be substituted and first generation cephalosporins are also effective. Tetracyclines should not be used for streptococcal infections.

Resistance of *Streptococcus pyogenes* to penicillins has not been reported. When patients do not respond clinically to treatment, lack of compliance or a mixed infection should be suspected.

Acute glomerulonephritis (AGN) may follow streptococcal infection by nephritogenic strains particularly in children. Early recognition of increased incidence of AGN in a community, and institution of public health measures, may prevent this complication from reaching epidemic proportions. Unlike streptococcal pharyngitis, streptococcal skin infections are not associated with rheumatic fever.

STAPHYLOCOCCAL INFECTIONS

Folliculitis

Clinical features   This is a relatively mild infection of hair follicles, usually by strains of *Staph. aureus* common on normal skin. A pustular eruption is produced in hairy areas including scalp, beard, axillae, trunk and buttocks. It is more prevalent in hot climates, particularly on occluded skin in obese persons or, for example, on the the buttocks in subjects sitting on plastic seats, or in persons wearing occlusive clothing (Fig. 1.3).

Management   Treatment consists of oral antibiotics to which the infecting strain is sensitive, and modification of the micro-environment to reduce occlusion and sweating. Total body bathing with chlorhexidine detergent cleansers on a daily basis until lesions clear, followed by twice weekly bathing reduces the total load of *Staph. aureus* on the skin and often prevents recurrence.

Furunculosis (boils)

Clinical features   This is a more severe infection of hair follicles resulting in painful subcutaneous abscesses. It is caused by more virulent strains of *Staph. aureus*, which are usually resistant to beta-lactamase degradeable

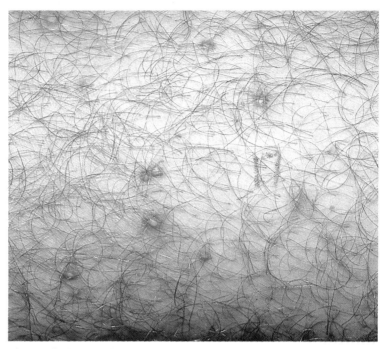

Fig. 1.3 Occlusive clothes in a hot climate contributed to this staphylococcal folliculitis.

penicillins and often to tetracyclines. Recurrent furunculosis, particularly in the crural area and buttocks, may be related to intimate contact with another person.

Management Oral cloxacillin, dicloxacillin or flucloxacillin are the preferred drugs. First generation cephalosporins and erythromycin are also effective.

Treatment should be instituted promptly on an empirical basis. Initial bacteriological samples will provide an accurate guide for antibiotic treatment and early treatment of contacts who may develop boils.

Large, painful furuncles may require incision and drainage (Fig. 1.4). This may be avoided by early treatment. The purulent exudate from furuncles which rupture spontaneously, or following incision, is a potent source of re-infection and transmission to others. In recurrent folliculitis or furunculosis the presence of a nasal carriage state should be suspected and if present treated with an antibacterial cream applied to the external nares.

Staphylococcal bullous impetigo

Clinical features This is caused by strains of *Staph. aureus* which elicit exfoliatin, an enzyme which produces cleavage in the upper layer of the epidermis. Common sites are the peri-oral area, nares, ears and axillae (Fig. 1.5). Lesions begin as small vesicles which rapidly spread to form clusters of pus filled bullae. On rupture, a thin, sticky, honey-coloured crust forms.

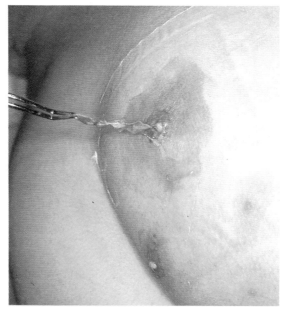

Fig. 1.4   The painful procedure of incision and drainage can be avoided by early treatment of boils.

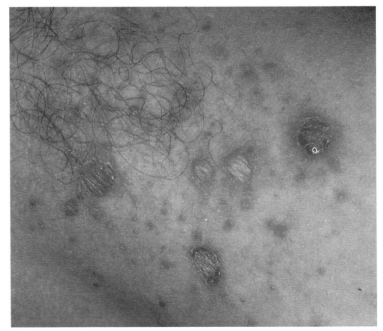

Fig. 1.5   Staphylococcal bullous impetigo.

Lesions rarely become echthymatous, except when secondarily infected with *Streptococcus pyogenes*. Outbreaks may occur among young schoolchildren and, occasionally, in adults requiring epidemiologic control measures.

Management Treatment is to remove the crusts with warm olive oil and to apply a topical antibacterial. Systemic antibiotics may also be needed. Topical antibiotics may be useful in preventing infections of clean wounds and probably reduce the chances of reinfection and transmission to others. They appear to have little advantage over gentle debridement and clean, light dressings, once the lesions are established and crusted. Neomycin and thiomerosal preparations may produce allergic reactions. Chlorhexidine gluconate cleansers used prophylactically reduce the bacterial load on the skin and are effective against staphylococci and streptococci.

Staphylococcal scalded skin syndrome
(toxic epidermal necrolysis or SSSS)

Clinical features This is a more dramatic expression of infection by exfoliatin–producing strains of *Staph. aureus*. It occurs mainly in infants and young children in whom large areas of skin become denuded, giving the appearance of red, moist, scalded skin (Fig. 1.6). It follows a primary impetigo and may be considered as a generalized reaction to the exfoliatin. Cultures from denuded areas are negative.

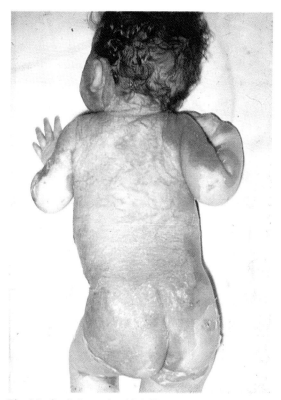

Fig. 1.6 Staphylococcal scalded skin syndrome.

Management

Prompt treatment with systemic anti-staphylococcal antibiotics is indicated. Hospitalization is the rule and appropriate measures must be taken to combat fluid, electrolyte and protein imbalance and to correct thermoregulatory dysfunction. Steroid therapy is contraindicated in SSSS.

GRAM-NEGATIVE INFECTIONS

Pseudomonas infections

Clinical features

Pseudomonas aeruginosa remains the most important Gram-negative organism causing cutaneous infections. Considered an opportunistic organism, it rarely invades healthy skin except under unusual conditions. It continues to pose a threat to patients with burns, diabetes or immunodeficiency.

Pseudomonas aeruginosa may cause otitis externa, toe web infections, necrotizing ulcers, green nails, corneal ulceration and a generalized folliculitis associated with hot tubs and whirlpool baths.

Toxin and enzyme production varies between strains, as does individual host susceptibility, so that it is difficult to predict the course of infection in an individual patient.

In general, the number of bacteria per surface area or gram of tissue is related to the severity of tissue destruction. Because this bacterium requires moist or wet conditions to thrive, removal of aqueous sources, alleviation of skin occlusion and drying measures will do much to prevent colonization and multiplication.

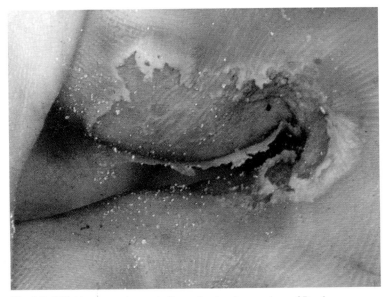

Fig. 1.7 This blue green pigment indicates the abundant presence of *Pseudomonas aeruginosa* in a toe web infection.

Heavy colonization of burns, ulcers, toe webs and dermatoses can be detected under long-wave ultraviolet light (Wood's lamp). Colonized areas fluoresce aqua green. This method may also be used to detect colonies of *Pseudomonas aeruginosa* on blood agar plates. Visible green or bluish-green pigment is also a useful diagnostic sign (Fig. 1.7) but the absence of fluorescence or visible pigment does not rule out infection.

A well-defined pseudomonal rash has been associated with use of hot tubs and whirlpool baths. It is identified by recent (24−48 hrs) history of immersion in a hot tub or whirlpool bath, and the appearance of a maculopapular, pustular rash on the trunk, axillae and buttocks. Systemic signs may include malaise, lymphadenopathy, fever, tender breasts, nausea, cramps and vomiting.

Pseudomonas aeruginosa infections of the nail and paronychia are often associated with wet occupations and frequently are accompanied by *Candida albicans*. Cultures are often negative by the time patients are seen but the disease is clearly associated with *Pseudomonas aeruginosa*.

Management

The rash, associated with whirlpool baths, is usually self-limiting in 1−2 weeks. Symptomatic therapy and attention to the offending water source is generally all that is required. Bromine-based water treatment is more effective than those based on chlorine.

Superficial infections of the toe webs may be improved by less occlusive footwear and drying agents, such as 5−10% aluminium chloride solution. Primary irritation and stinging may occur in open fissures or denuded skin.

Pseudomonas infections of the nails and paronychia are treated with drying agents, such as alcohol. Topical antifungals with topical steroids are helpful but a change of occupation may be necessary to effect a cure. Use of lined plastic or rubber gloves for dishwashing is advised.

Silver sulphadiazine cream is widely used for prevention of pseudonomas infections in burns. Systemic therapy for *Pseudomonas aeruginosa* should be guided by the antibiotic sensitivity of the strain(s). Careful monitoring is indicated during therapy with aminoglycoside antibiotics to avoid ototoxicity and nephrotoxicity.

Other Gram-negative infections

Clinical features

Gram-negative folliculitis is a complication of acne vulgaris occurring most often in patients receiving long-term tetracycline therapy. A variety of lactose fermenting bacteria are associated with the pustular form, which is the most common presentation. A devastating foul smelling cystic and nodular form is associated with Proteus species.

Management

Long-term therapy with ampicillin or co-trimoxazole is indicated in Gram-negative folliculitis and antibiotic sensitivities should be obtained.

FUNGAL INFECTIONS

Dermatophytosis (ringworm)

Clinical features   These are superficial infections of the stratum corneum, hair and nails by dermatophilic fungi which cause inflammatory responses in the host. Anthropophilic species, such as *Trichophyton rubrum* and *Epidermophyton flocossum* have become adapted to man, and are responsible for most human infections. Zoophilic species, of which *Microsporum canis* and certain strains of *Trichophyton mentagrophytes* are examples, have their natural reservoir in animals but occasionally infect man.

Geophilic species include the soil-inhabiting fungi with keratinophilic properties, such as *Microsporum gypseum*. These are responsible for rare infections in gardeners, farmers and others who are in contact with plants or soil. Extra-human species usually cause acute, highly inflammatory, often discrete lesions on exposed surfaces. Anthropophilic infections may be chronic, with minimal signs of inflammation.

The degree of cutaneous reaction to the antigens and extracellular products of fungal metabolism vary considerably and are modified by the immunologic status of the host, previous encounters with the infecting strains and environmental temperature.

Occlusion and sweating play a significant role in exacerbating quiescent infections and the extent and severity of new infections. Occluded body sites are the most commonly affected and include the toe webs (Fig. 1.8), inner thighs, buttocks and axillae in men (Fig. 1.9). Although dermatophytosis is relatively rare in women, the condition may occur under pendulous breasts, axillae and inner thighs in the obese and in women wearing occlusive shoes.

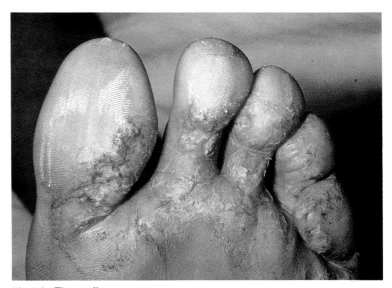

Fig. 1.8   Tinea pedis.

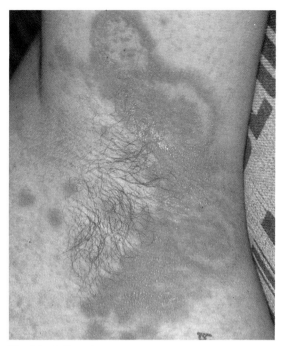

Fig. 1.9   Axillary ringworm.

Typical lesions of the glabrous skin are red, pruritic and scaly. The advancing border is well defined and may show tiny vesicles. As the border advances, older areas heal and may appear almost normal. This phenomenon may result in circinate lesions, hence the term 'ringworm' (Fig. 1.9).

Two types of fungi infect the scalp. Certain Microsporum species form an aggregation of spores around hair shafts (ectothrix) and produce a green fluorescence under long-wave ultra violet light (Wood's lamp). These infections often produce patches of alopecia. Trichophyton species invade the hair shaft (endothrix) and produce a diffuse, scaling folliculitis. Hairs may break off under the skin surface, producing a 'chicken skin' appearance. These do not fluoresce with Wood's lamp.

Diagnosis of dermatophytosis is made on clinical grounds and confirmed by microscopical examination of superficial skin scrapings cleared in 20% potassium hydroxide solution. Scrapings are best made from the roofs of vesicles and active borders of lesions. Infected hairs may be plucked with forceps.

Confirmation of infecting species is made by culture of scrapings made on selective media for fungi. Dermatophyte Test Media (DTM) can be used by those without access to a laboratory.

Management   Removal of occlusive clothing and footwear, change of occupation or relocation to a cooler climate are important considerations in the management of dermatophytosis.

Most cases of dermatophytosis on glabrous skin can be managed by topical therapy and appropriate measures to relieve occlusion. Creams and lotions containing imidazoles are effective against dermatophyte fungi and *Candida albicans*. Useful agents include clotrimazole, econazole, miconazole and sulconazole. Ciclopirox olamine is a non-imidazole topical anti-fungal agent which is also effective against dermatophyte fungi and *Candida albicans*. A single application at night to the infected area is as effective as twice-daily therapy. Combinations of topical antifungal creams and a medium potency topical steroid more rapidly alleviate itching and erythema but steroid creams alone should never be used on fungal or candidal infections. Tolnaftate is an effective antidermatophytic agent, but has no effect on candidosis. Topical nystatin is not effective for dermatophytosis. Powders containing antifungal agents may have some effect in preventing exacerbation or acquisition of fungal infections but are relatively ineffective for treatment of well-established lesions.

Infections of hair and nails respond to oral griseofulvin (see Ch. 20). 500 mg per day of the microcrystalline form is recommended for tinea corporis, cruris and capitis. 250 mg per day for children under 50 lbs is usually adequate. Tinea pedis and infections of the nails may require double the above doses. Treatment is continued until clinical signs and fungal cultures are negative and range from 3−4 weeks for tinea corporis or up to a year for obstinate infections of toenails. The drug should be taken with a fatty meal.

Candidosis

Clinical features   This is infection of occluded skin and mucous membranes by the yeast *Candida albicans*. It is more common in diabetics, pregnant women and obese persons and is a common cause of vulvo-vaginitis and severe

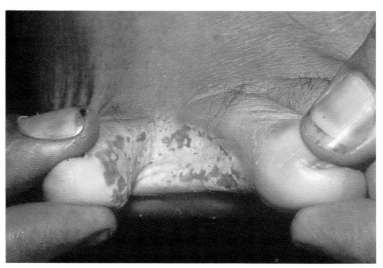

Fig. 1.10   Thickened white stratum corneum and small patches of denudation are typical of candidosis in intertriginous sites.

napkin rash in infants, particularly in tropical climates. Oral antibiotics may alter the ecology of the gut flora, allowing overgrowth of *Candida albicans* which may proceed to perianal dermatitis, crural candidosis and vulvo-vaginitis. Diagnosis may be confirmed by potassium hydroxide preparations, Gram's stain and culture.

The lesions are bright red, or even denuded, and often exhibit 'satellite' pustules. They are intensely pruritic. In intertriginous areas, or under the foreskin, white macerated skin with islands of bright red denudation are typical (Fig. 1.10).

Chronic candida paronychia (see Ch. 20)

Management

Management involves alleviation of occlusion and topical therapy with broad spectrum imidazole agents other than ketoconazole or with ciclopirox olamine. Oral nystatin may be administered to reduce colonization of the gut when this is the source, and the daily administration of *Lactobacillus acidophilus* or unpasteurized yoghurt will assist in re-establishing normal flora. Widespread, severe or recurrent candidosis should invite a suspicion of diabetes. Topical nystatin preparations are also effective.

In vulvo-vaginal candidosis, nystatin pessaries or imidazole creams are standard therapy. Avoidance of occlusive underwear, pantyhose and tight jeans do much to alleviate this common and troublesome problem. In severe and extensive cases not responsive to other therapy systemic ketoconazole may be required (see Ch. 22).

Tinea versicolor (pityriasis versicolor)

Clinical features

This is superficial infection of the stratum corneum by the yeast *Pityrosporum orbiculare*. Small to confluent, slightly scaly patches of depigmentation are produced usually on the back, chest, upper arms, neck or face. Usually these are not highly inflammatory or symptomatic (Fig. 1.11). The yeast produces an extracellular substance which interferes with normal pigmentation. Lesions often become apparent after suntanning, giving rise to the lay term 'sun fungus'. Diagnosis is confirmed by microscopic examination of scrapings, which reveal typical spores and short hyphae.

Management

Management consists of topical application of selenium sulphide shampoo, which is lathered over the head and trunk, left to dry overnight, and rinsed off the next morning. Three consecutive nights' treatment are usually sufficient.

Shampoos containing 2% sulphur and 2% salicylic acid have also been reported to be effective. A simple remedy consists of 50% propylene glycol solution, applied at night for 2 weeks. It is mildly keratolytic and has antifungal properties. Avoidance of eyes and genitalia is advised for the above remedies. Topical miconazole and sodium hyposulphite are

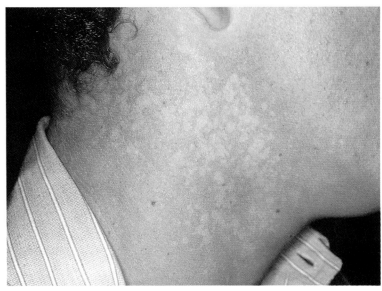

Fig. 1.11 Tinea versicolor.

also recommended remedies. The organism is sensitive to ketoconazole but this should only be used in severe resistant cases.

VIRAL INFECTIONS

Herpes simplex

Clinical features *Herpes simplex type 1* may affect any site in the body. Primary infection in childhood may present as a severe herpetic stomatitis with systemic signs. The disease may be recurrent in one site at intervals varying from weeks to years. Characteristically, the lesions start with itching; small turbid vesicles rapidly develop (Fig. 1.12). These vesicles rupture and crusts are formed. Untreated, the lesion heals in 7–10 days.

Herpes simplex type 2 affect the genital mucosa almost exclusively. The clinical history is the same as for *Herpes simplex type 1.*

Management Two antiviral agents are used: idoxuridine (IDU) as a 5% solution in Dimethyl sulphoxide (DMSO) and acyclovir in a cream base. The latter can also be used if the eye is involved. Recurrent herpes simplex can be treated with the same agents. Some believe that superficial X-ray therapy (800 R at 10 kV) reduces the frequency of the attacks. Secondary infection is common and may require systemic antibiotics. Children with atopic eczema must be protected from contact with *Herpes simplex* virus. The acquisition of the virus in these children results in a generalised herpetic infection (eczema herpeticum) with a high morbidity and potential mortality.

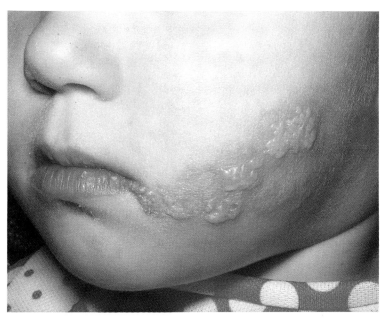

Fig. 1.12   Herpes simplex.

Herpes zoster (shingles)

Clinical features   Infection by the *Varicella zoster* virus results in a dermatomal distribution of painful haemorrhagic vesicles (Fig. 1.13). Its occurrence in multiple dermatomes suggest underlying immunodeficiency.

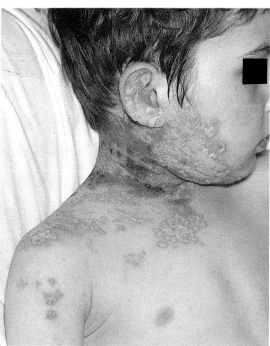

Fig. 1.13   Herpes zoster (note haemorrhagic nature of blisters).

Management   To be effective antiviral agents need to be used within hours of the vesicles developing. Idoxuridine and acyclovir topically have some effect. A major problem is the occurrence of post-herpetic neuralgia in the elderly. Prevention may be hoped for by treatment with systemic corticosteroids or acyclovir (see Ch. 22). Analgesics will be required for the pain.

Warts

Clinical features   There are many clinical varieties of warts and at least six wart viruses have been identified. Common warts may appear on the hands, face or almost any part of the body. Plantar warts, by definition, appear on the soles of the feet. Recurrence of genital warts, especially in adults, should lead to investigation of any sexual partners and many believe that all patients with such warts should be investigated by venereologists. Molluscum contagiosum due to a very large virus occurs predominantly in children and may be a major problem in atopics.

Warts in general are a problem in immunocompromised patients, either due to therapy or disease.

Management   Common warts are best left alone in children as most of them disappear spontaneously in 12−18 months. If treatment is required, salicylic acid, lactic acid or gluteraldehyde preparations are useful. In the older child or the adult cryotherapy with liquid nitrogen is very successful. Warts in beard areas in males and on the lips are best treated by curettage and cauterisation.

Periungual warts constitute a particular problem and are best treated by a local preparation as described above, under adhesive plaster for 3 days at a time.

Genital warts can be treated with 10−25% podophyllin in spirit, painted on and then washed off thoroughly in 6 hours. Cryotherapy and curretage are often needed if podophyllin fails.

Molluscum contagiosum in children can be treated by applications of salicylic acid as discussed above. Sodium fusidate ointment is often used but whether or not it has any action on the virus is not clear at present. Solitary or small numbers of lesions can be treated by 'spiking' with a sharpened orange stick dipped in liquid phenol or 40% trichloracetic acid.

The management of warts is full of many anecdotal treatments and, strangely, hypnosis may result in their resolution if they are very extensive or persistent.

Orf

Clinical features   This is an ulcerative stomatitis of sheep which can be transmitted to man by direct contact with the infected animal or from occupational contact such as by a butcher from a sheep's head. The disease is due to a virus of the paravaccinia group. The characteristic lesion is an inflamed violaceous nodule which can reach 1–2 cm in diameter and can be very tender (Fig. 1.14).

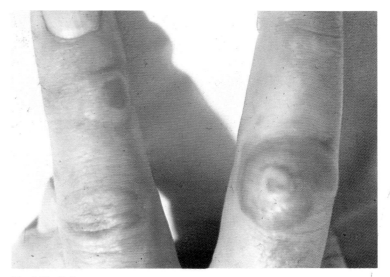

Fig. 1.14 Orf.

Management   The lesions are often incised in error but if the clinical diagnosis is made, the patient should be managed conservatively. Topical antibiotics may be required. Cellulitis surrounding the lesion may occur and this will require systemic antibiotics.

Hand, foot and mouth disease

Clinical features   This is due to Coxsackie virus infection and is characterised by small blisters on hands, feet and oral mucosa. It occurs in epidemics and may give rise to little systemic effect.

Management   This is conservative but mouth lesions may require soothing mouthwashes (see Formulary).

FURTHER READING

Blankenship M L 1984 Gram-negative folliculitis. Archives of Dermatology 120: 1301
Chandrasekar P H, Rolston K V I, Kannangara W, Le Frock J L, Binnick, S A 1984
    Hot tub-associated dermatitis due to *Pseudomonas aeruginosa* Archives of Dermatology
    120: 1337
Noble W C 1983 Microbial skin disease: its epidemiology. Edward Arnold, London and
    Baltimore.
Noble W C, Rook A 1981 Microbiology of human skin: major problems in dermatology
    Lloyd-Luke (Medical Books) Ltd., London, U.K.
Schachner L, Taplin D, Scott G B, Morrison M 1983 A therapeutic update of
    superficial skin infections. Pediatric Clinics of North America 30(2): 397

D. Taplin

2. Cutaneous Infestatations

SCABIES

Clinical features This is a pruritic maculo-papular, pustular eruption caused by the burrowing of the female mite Sarcoptes scabiei var hominis.

Nocturnal itching, typical body distribution and evidence of contact transmission to or from others provide a provisional diagnosis. Definitive diagnosis is made by finding the mite or eggs of the mite in superficial skin scrapings (Fig. 2.1). A drop of mineral oil is placed on a suspected lesion or burrow and scraped vigorously with a scalpel. The scrapings and oil are examined with a powerful hand lens or low-power microscope. The acarus may also be picked out with the point of a blind pin.

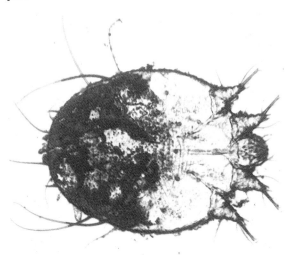

Fig. 2.1 Mineral oil mount of the female scabies mite.

In adults, lesions are found in the finger webs, flexor surfaces of wrists, extensor surfaces of elbows, axillary folds, gluteal cleft, areolae of breasts and under the breasts in women, and on the penile shaft in men. Palms, soles and face are usually spared. In tropical areas, large areas of the chest and abdomen may be involved in infants and in women wearing occlusive clothing. In young children and infants, particularly in warm climates, scabies lesions may be found on palms and soles, neck and behind the ears. Infants often develop infiltrated nodular lesions in the axillae (Fig. 2.2). Burrows are more common in cooler climates and quite rare in the tropics where lesions often appear as 1–2 mm red papules.

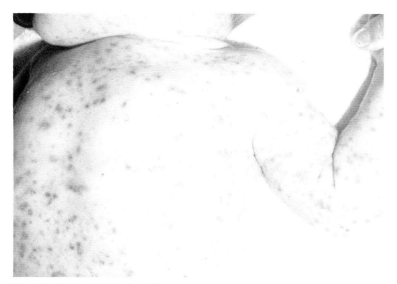

Fig. 2.2 Nodules in infantile scabies.

Two enhancement techniques have been developed which make burrows easier to find. The Cullen and Childers method utilizes 0.5% tetracycline solution, made by adding 500 mg of tetracycline to 20 ml glycerin, made up to 100 ml with absolute ethanol. The solution is applied to the suspected area of skin and allowed to dry for 5 minutes. The skin is wiped vigorously with isopropanol, leaving residual tetracycline in the burrow which can be detected as golden yellow fluorescence under Wood's light. The Burrow Ink Test utilizes black or blue ink, or felt pen in the same fashion. Burrows can be seen in visible light. Colour illustrations of these and other diagnostic aids are shown in an excellent monograph by Estes. Mites, eggs or their remnants may be found under the fingernails.

Management   The most widely prescribed treatment for scabies is 1% gamma benzene hexachloride (lindane) lotion. A single head-to-toe application for 8–12 hours is usually sufficient and all close contacts should always be treated concurrently whether or not they exhibit active infestation, since they may be in the incubation stage. In high density populations, refugee camps or similar situations of overcrowding, treatment of individual cases is wasteful of time and medication, since they will invariably become reinfested.

Lindane preparations should be used with caution, since there is a potential for CNS toxicity following cutaneous absorption. This is particularly true in infants (see Ch. 13).

10% crotamiton is an antipruritic lotion with reputed antiscabietic properties. Clinical response is poor and the requirement for multiple treatments over several days severely limits its value. Toxicity data on crotamiton is meagre.

5% precipitated sulphur in soft paraffin is of value for use on children, and sulphur has been used for over 2000 years for the 'itch'. Application for three consecutive nights is recommended. The formulation is messy, may stain clothing and has an objectionable odour. In hot climates, irritation in intertriginous areas may occur.

In many countries, 25% benzyl benzoate emulsion is used. It should be applied on two consecutive nights following a bath.

Secondary bacterial infections of scabies are extremely common in tropical climates. Concurrent systemic treatment for streptococcal/ staphylococcal infections is indicated and a second treatment with the topical scabiecide may be necessary after the skin infections have healed.

Sarcoptes scabiei var hominis and the dog mite (var canis) can survive up to 36 hours away from the host at room temperatures and humidities. Survival is even longer at lower temperatures. Treatment of bed linens and clothing by hot water and hot drying cycles is, therefore, advisable. Clothing which cannot be heated should be dry cleaned. Environmental sprays containing synergized pyrethrins or synthetic pyrethroids are available commercially for disinfesting furniture and mattresses.

PEDICULOSIS

Pediculosis capitis

Clinical features This is an infestation of the scalp area by Pediculus humanus var capitis, the human head louse. These blood sucking, wingless insects utilize human blood as their sole source of nutrition and obtain it by thrusting a pair of stylets through the epidermis, producing microscopic lacerations. Saliva, thought to contain anticoagulants, is injected which produces pruritus.

In heavily infested individuals, several hundred bites are inflicted daily. Clinical signs vary from erythematous, macular, excoriated, highly pruritic skin to no visible reactions at all. Both hypersensitivity and acquired tolerance are, therefore, encountered. The female head louse is fertilized five or six times a day and lays eggs which she firmly cements to the hair shaft with a substance which has so far eluded analysis.

In temperate climates, most eggs are laid within 1 cm of the scalp. In tropical humid climates, new viable eggs may be found at random on the hair but the majority are still found close to the scalp. In 7–10 days, the eggs hatch into colourless nymphs, about 0.5 mm long. Following three moults, the lice become fertile adults in 2–3 weeks, and the cycle is repeated. Adult lice are reddish brown to dark mahogany in colour and 2–2.5 mm long (Fig. 2.3). Fertile eggs are 0.7 mm long and 0.3 mm in diameter, tan to dark brown in colour. Following hatching, the empty egg case, or nit, remains attached to the hair, and is pale or white in colour.

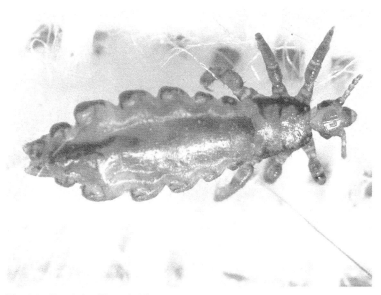

Fig. 2.3   Female head louse (x 15).

Pediculosis capitis is not associated with poor hygiene or neglect. It is rare among curly haired black children in the USA but may be found in straight haired Asian, Hispanic and Caucasian subjects.

Transmission occurs primarily by close contact. This is thought to be the reason for the higher prevalence in young children who make frequent contact during play. Human head lice cannot remain off the human host for more than 10 hours without a blood meal. Eggs on shed hairs remain viable until hatching under favourable temperature and humidity. They are a potential source of infestation. In cool climates, environmental reservoirs are not considered likely sources of infestation.

Management   Management of pediculosis capitis varies with availability of pesticides in different countries. These include 1% lindane shampoo, 0.5% malathion lotion, products based on natural pyrethrins synergized with piperonyl butoxide and carbaryl containing pesticides.

1% lindane shampoo continues to be effective in the USA but resistance to head and body lice has been reported from several countries.

Lindane shampoo is not completely ovicidal since 30% or more of the eggs survive treatment. A second treatment 7−10 days later may be necessary to kill the young nymphs from surviving eggs and is unlikely to induce CNS toxicity in healthy subjects. Use of lindane in underweight, malnourished or otherwise compromised children is ill-advised.

Malathion lotion is a highly effective pesticide and ovicide. The alcoholic vehicle is flammable and malathion is malodorous. These characteristics, and high cost, limit patient acceptance. Malathion is less toxic than lindane, and CNS toxicity has not been reported. Synergized pyrethrins are effective but like lindane shampoo, are not completely ovicidal. A second treatment 7−10 days later is advised. Mammalian toxicity is low and CNS toxicity is not known to occur.

Carbaryl shampoo 0.5% is an effective pediculicide but is not completely ovicidal and a second treatment is recommended.

Pediculosis corporis

Clinical features

Infestation of clothing and bedding by Pediculus humanus, the human body louse or, more accurately, the clothing louse.

Unlike pediculosis capitis, this is a disease of the vagabonds, derelicts and refugees of society. The insect causing the disease lives in clothing but, like the other lice of man, derives its sole nourishment from human blood. It is somewhat hardier than its cousin, the head louse, and less dependent on frequent blood meals. Except when feeding, it resides in clothing, and lays its eggs in the seams of the crotch, armpit, beltline and neckband.

Although lice are rarely found on the body, the signs of their presence are readily seen. These may include vertical excoriations of trunk, thighs and buttocks, hyperpigmented macules and post-inflammatory hyperpigmentation and lichenification resulting from frequent scratching of this highly pruritic affliction. Victims are usually encountered in emergency rooms, street clinics and public health facilities.

Management

Management often consists of destruction of clothing by burning, a hot bath and total body application of 1% lindane lotion. Referral to social services may be instituted to rescue the subject from the living conditions associated with body lice.

In many areas of the world, such luxuries are unavailable or prohibitively costly. In these situations, and particularly during war and famine, large scale delousing with dusting powders is employed to prevent or halt epidemics of serious diseases such as louse-borne typhus, relapsing fever and trench fever. Pesticides which have been used in dusting powders include carbaryl, DDT, lindane, malathion, permethrin, propoxur and temephos. Unfortunately, resistance of body lice to DDT, dieldrin and lindane is now widespread, and resistance to malathion has been reported.

Pediculosis pubis

Clinical features

This is an infestation of the pubic, and occasionally other hairy areas of the body, by Phthirus pubis, the crab louse (Fig. 2.4). Like the other human lice, these insects feed only on human blood.

Diagnosis is usually made by the patient, who develops pruritus, and one day makes the horrifying discovery of small (1–1.5 mm) brown creatures crawling in the pubic area. On examination with a hand lens, they do indeed look like tiny crabs. Rarely, bluish macules are seen on the skin and are considered to be characteristic. They are caused by conversion of haemoglobin to biliverdin by enzymes in the saliva of the insect.

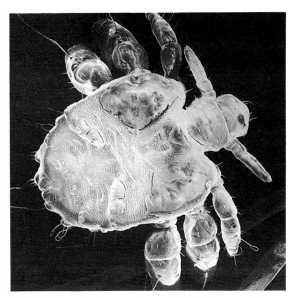

Fig. 2.4 Scanning electron micrograph of the human crab louse.

Tan to dark brown eggs, somewhat smaller than those of head lice are found cemented to the pubic hairs, and in older infestations, the whitish transluscent empty nits may be mistaken for seborrheic scales (dandruff). The emotional effects associated with discovery of these new found friends are immediate and impressive, and there is no doubt that many infestations are promptly dealt with by a fast trip to the nearest pharmacy.

Intimate contact with another person is the most efficient means of transmission and there is no doubt that pubic lice may be acquired during sexual activity. This is by no means the only source, since live Phthirus pubis have been found on towels, toilet seats and beds. Occasionally, they may occur in other hairy areas, including the eyelashes. In children, the eyelashes may be the only site involved, most likely because the grasping claws of the crab louse are shaped to fit stout, oval section hairs.

The shedding of hairs with viable eggs represents another potential mode of transmission. Many a travelling celibate has been unjustly accused of misbehaviour when his only misfortune was to sleep in a recently occupied hotel room. Nevertheless, once the diagnosis is made, current or recent contacts should also be treated to avoid reinfestation.

Management A variety of synergized pyrethrin products are available which are effective, and should be used twice, the second application 7–10 days after the first treatment, to kill nymphs hatched from eggs not affected by the first application. The older practice of shaving the area is not necessary.

Hot laundering of bedding, clothes and towels is advised. Mattresses and furniture may be sprayed with commercially available synergized pyrethrins or pyrethroids.

Management of pediculosis pubis is the same as for head lice, with the exception of alcoholic malathion lotion, which is not recommended for use in the pubic area.

Treatment of crab lice in the eyebrows or eyelashes presents problems, since products intended for pediculosis may produce eye irritation. Soft paraffin applied twice daily for a week, with mechanical removal of eggs, is reported to be effective.

Papular urticaria (Lichen urticatus)

Clinical features

This is a very common condition especially in children and it is often called 'heat spots'. Characteristically crops of urticarial lesions arise on the trunk and limbs. These may blister and they are intensely pruritic (Fig. 2.5). They rapidly become excoriated (Fig. 2.6), are often secondarily infected and heal leaving characteristic pigmented scars.

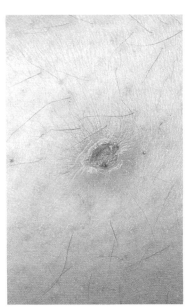

Fig. 2.6 Excoriation in papular urticaria.

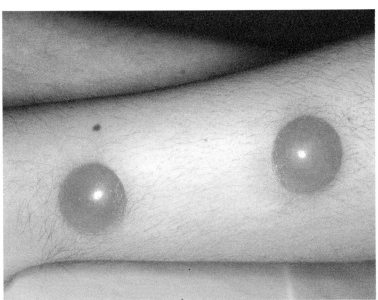

Fig. 2.5 Bullae in papular urticaria.

Innumerable insects cause this problem: dog fleas, cat fleas and cheyletiella. Almost all pet animals carry mites capable of producing this condition. Investigation is by obtaining brushings from bedding, clothing and family pets for microscopic examination.

Management

The management is the identification of the offending mite and its eradication by suitable pesticides, usually pyrethrum or malathion. Gamma benzene hexachloride is also useful. The pesticide should be applied to the animal carrier, to bedding, soft furniture and the outer inch of fitted carpets. Local treatment of the patient with antipruritics such as Calamine Lotion with 1% phenol and with systemic antihistamines is indicated.

FURTHER READING

Eaglestein W H, Pariser D M 1978 Office techniques for diagnosing skin disease. Year book, Medical Publishers, Chicago

Estes S A 1981 The diagnosis and management of scabies. Obtainable from the Department of Dermatology, University of Cincinnati Medical Center, Cincinnati, Ohio

Maunders J W 1983 The appreciation of lice. Proceedings of the Royal Institute of Great Britain 55 Chameleon Press, London

Woodley D, Saurat J H 1981 The Burrow Ink Test and the scabies mite. Journal of the American Academy of Dermatology 4: 715

Alan R. Shalita

3. Acne Vulgaris, Rosacea, Disorders of the Sweat Glands

ACNE VULGARIS

Clinical features

The most common disease of the cutaneous appendages is acne vulgaris. Often mistakenly referred to as a disease of the sebaceous glands, acne is really a disease of the pilosebaceous unit. The sebaceous glands are stimulated by androgens to increase in size and output of sebum. Sebum stimulates abnormal follicular keratinization, or comedogenesis, and provides an excellent environment for the proliferation of *Propionibacterium acnes*. Products secreted by *P. acnes* contribute to further changes in the follicular epithelium which result in comedo formation. Other products of *P. acnes* are chemotactic to leukocytes and initiate inflammation.

Acne usually begins with a few comedones on or about the nose or forehead. Mild forms remain primarily comedonal with relatively few lesions and an occasional inflammatory papule. In the more typical case, more open and closed comedones are present, with 10–20 inflammatory papules and/or pustules. In more severe disease inflammatory lesions predominate, although there may also be many comedones (Fig. 3.1). There may be an occasional nodulocystic lesion and the shoulders may become involved. Acne is very severe when nodulocystic lesions are more numerous and/or the back and chest are significantly affected (Fig. 3.2). When lesions coalesce to become multilobular with sinus tracts and double comedones, then it is termed Acne Conglobata.

Management

The common denominator in all acne is the microcomedo, the precursor of both open and closed comedones (blackheads and whiteheads) and of inflammatory lesions such as papules, pustules and cysts. So it is logical to start treatment with topically applied tretinoin, the only drug which significantly reduces microcomedo formation. Since topical tretinoin may be highly irritating, particularly to individuals with fair skin, it is wise to initiate therapy with the mildest form, then increase the concentration or change the vehicle as tolerated. Some may need treatment on alternate days before they can tolerate daily dosage. Common side-effects are erythema, peeling and increased sensitivity to ultra-violet light. If these side-effects are carefully explained and appropriate precautions taken, patient compliance is enhanced and rewarding results may be expected.

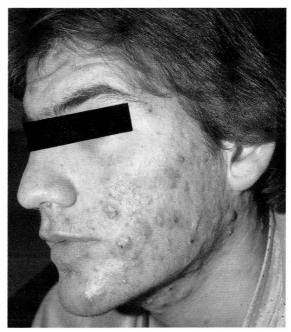

Fig. 3.1 Pustules and other inflammatory acne lesions in adults (note tendency of lesions to localize along mandible and on neck).

A second popular and logical treatment is the use of topical antibacterial agents which reduce the follicular population of *P. acnes*. They include topical formulations of benzoyl peroxide and of broad spectrum antibiotics such as erythromycin and clindamycin. Benzoyl peroxide is a potent oxidizing agent which effectively reduces *P. acnes* populations in skin. It may possess mild comedolytic activity. It is particularly effective in mild to moderate cases of inflammatory acne with counts of papules and pustules usually falling by 50–75%. Benzoyl peroxide often causes skin irritation and, occasionally, allergic eczematous contact dermatitis. If therapy is started cautiously with low concentrations or low irritancy vehicles, then one may progress to stronger concentrations and/or vehicles.

Topical antibiotics are frequently useful as an alternative to benzoyl peroxide when the latter is not well tolerated due to irritation or sensitization. In general, the results are similar to those achieved with benzoyl peroxide but certainly not superior. Although usually well tolerated, topical antibiotics may lose their efficacy because resistant strains of *P. acnes* develop. After a rest, the sensitive strains invariably return. Extensive clinical use in the USA suggests that the development of resistant organisms other than *P. acnes* is not a significant clinical problem. It is now common to use one or more combinations of these agents in acne. The sequential use of tretinoin and benzoyl peroxide or tretinoin and a topical antibiotic, one in the morning and the other in the evening, is more effective than either agent used alone. One proprietary preparation successfully combines tretinoin with a topical antibiotic.

Similarly, benzoyl peroxide and topical antibiotics may be used sequentially to advantage. A combined formulation of benzoyl peroxide and erythromycin is more effective than either ingredient alone.

Painful, tense inflammatory lesions (Fig. 3.2) may be lanced with the point of a scalpel or a large bore needle and the contents expressed. Alternatively, they may be successfully treated by intralesional injection of triamcinolone acetonide, 2.5–5.0 mg/ml or its equivalent. Local atrophy may be avoided by injecting small amounts (0.1 ml) at low concentration. This treatment rapidly resolves inflammatory lesions.

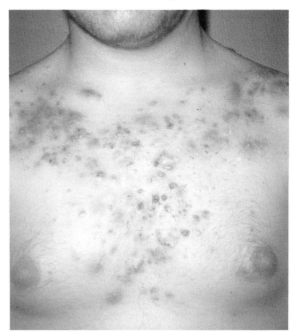

Fig. 3.2   Inflammatory acne of chest.

Visible comedones may be removed with a comedo extractor. This removes unsightly lesions and helps the patient to comply with the rest of the treatment since he or she sees the immediate results.

In spite of the very effective topical treatment available, many more severe cases of acne need systemic antibiotics for adequate control. Tetracycline remains the drug of choice, although some of its derivatives, such as minocycline, may achieve higher tissue levels at lower dose. Tetracycline is usually given as 1 g/day in divided doses on an empty stomach and not with milk. After 1 month the dose may be either decreased or increased according to the therapeutic response. Many patients may be maintained on doses as low as 250–500 mg/day but some of the most severe cases may need as much as 3 g/day. Although tetracycline may be associated with numerous, unpleasant side-effects, patients have been followed for periods of 6 years or longer without significant deleterious effect.

Vaginitis due to *Candida albicans* is a common complication of therapy in women. It can usually be treated with local anti-candidal therapy without discontinuing the tetracycline, although that course may occasionally be necessary. Other side-effects include gastrointestinal upset, photosensitivity and non-specific dermatitis. In patients unable to take one of the tetracyclines, erythromycin is a satisfactory alternative, given in comparable doses.

HORMONES

Until recently, the only satisfactory method of reducing sebum production has been with systemic oestrogen therapy. Unfortunately, this has limited such treatment to women, although men may occasionally be treated successfully with low-dose glucocorticoids.

In women, the ovary and adrenal glands are sources of androgen. Ovarian androgen production may be suppressed with systemic oestrogen therapy, usually in the form of oral contraceptives. Although 100 mg of ethinyloestradiol or mestranol produce maximum inhibition of sebum production, lower doses are often prescribed in order to reduce side-effects. Combining oestrogen and the anti-androgen cyproterone acetate appears to be effective.

Glucocorticosteroids may be used to reduce adrenal androgen secretion, particularly in patients with a demonstrated increase in adrenal androgen production. Dexamethasone, 0.25−0.5 mg/day or prednisone 7.5−10.0 mg/day, appear to be effective. In some patients the glucocorticoids and oestrogens may be combined for maximal androgen inhibition. Suggestions that these low doses of glucocorticoids are also effective in men with increased adrenal androgen secretion, have yet to be confirmed.

In the most severe forms of inflammatory acne, higher doses of glucocorticosteroids such as prednisone, 40 mg/day, may be needed to control explosive flares of inflammatory lesions. Their use should be limited to 2−3 weeks to avoid serious sequellae.

ISOTRETINOIN

The most significant advance in acne treatment has been isotretinoin (13-cis retinoic acid) for severe, recalcitrant cystic acne. Although not common, cystic acne and acne conglobata are destructive, inflammatory variants which may cause physical and emotional scarring. Isotretinoin induces dramatic and prolonged remission of this most troublesome form of the disease. For dosages see Chapter 22. Patients with extensive disease of the trunk may need higher doses (up to 2 mg/kg/day). Lower doses, while effective, result in more frequent recurrence.

Isotretinoin has troublesome side-effects. It is teratogenic and must not be administered to pregnant women. The physician must be sure that the patient is not pregnant at start of treatment and that she practises strict contraception during treatment and for at least 1 month after it is complete. Isotretinoin is not mutagenic and does not affect human spermatogenesis.

The drug produces a profound, prolonged reduction in sebum production and in *P. acnes* counts. This dries the skin and mucous membranes to produce cheilitis and xerosis. Conjunctivitis and epistaxis and peeling of the palms and soles may also occur. Thinning of the hair is less common.

Among its systemic side-effects are transient elevation of liver enzymes and more persistent elevations of serum triglycerides. All return to normal after stopping treatment. There are rare reports of pseudotumour cerebrii, particularly if isotretinoin is used with tetracycline. Rarely, reversible corneal opacities have been reported. Hyperostoses occur in patients taking the drug in higher doses for longer periods than those recommended for acne. This toxicity profile should limit use of isotretinoin to recalcitrant cases of inflammatory acne which have failed to respond to adequate trials of conventional acne therapy, including systemic antibiotics (Fig. 3.2).

GRAM-NEGATIVE FOLLICULITIS

Clinical features Gram-negative folliculitis is a variant of acne resulting from over-growth of Gram-negative organisms. There are crops of pustules or nodules on the chin and perioral regions from which Gram-negative organisms are usually recovered. The organisms have usually travelled from the anterior nares, or the external ear in otitis externa.

Management Co-trimoxazole, two tablets twice daily, is very effective in many cases and the disease has been reported to respond dramatically to isotretinoin therapy in doses of 0.5 mg/kg for 1−2 months.

ROSACEA

Clinical features Rosacea or acne rosacea is an inflammatory disease of the facial skin. It is often associated with seborrhoea, but a cause and effect relationship has never been established. There is erythema, telangiectasia and occasionally, pustules. When more severe, it becomes granulomatous.

Management In most patients rosacea can be adequately controlled with long-term oral tetracyclines. The initial dose is 1g/day, switching quickly to a maintenance dose of 250−500 mg. Brief treatments with low-potency steroid creams or hydrocortisone and sulphur combined are useful. Prolonged topical steroid treatment, particularly of high potency, can produce rebound telangiectasia and aggravate the disease. Low doses of isotretinoin 0.2−0.5 mg/kg/day may dramatically improve the more severe forms of rosacea. Long-term follow-up, however, is not yet available.

HIDRADENITIS SUPPURATIVA

Clinical features

Hidradenitis suppurativa is a skin inflammation in areas where apocrine glands predominate, such as the axilla, groin and perianal region. It comprises abscess-like swelling, recurrent draining, secondary infection, then sinus formation and scarring.

Hidradenitis appears to be the result of occlusion of the apocrine and associated pilosebaceous ducts. The occluded ducts are an attractive environment for the proliferation of bacteria. Their rupture produces chemical and bacterial inflammation. Healing produces the scarring and sinus tracts. There is a chronic remission and exacerbation.

Management

Early management should be medical. Incising and draining the lesions often produces more complications than benefit. High doses of tetracyclines are frequently beneficial in the early stages. Lack of progress or failure to respond should lead to prompt culture of the draining material and then to the appropriate antibiotic. Much of the infection is in a sequestered site and higher than usual doses of antibiotics may be necessary. It is usual to initiate therapy with 1 g of a tetracycline/day and it may be necessary to increase this dose. Erythromycin in similar doses and co-trimoxazole, two tablets twice a day, are satisfactory alternatives.

In women, the disease may frequently be ameliorated by oral contraceptives. Oestrogen appears to reduce both sebaceous and apocrine gland activity. Isotretinoin helps but does not produce the dramatic and prolonged response seen in patients with cystic acne. A dose of 2 mg/kg/day is usually required and it should not be continued for longer than 20 weeks. Glucocorticosteroids, such as prednisone, in moderate doses for up to 2 weeks are of benefit against acute flares but should not be administered for long periods.

Simple incision and drainage is usually counterproductive, but intralesional corticosteroids may be most useful in controlling the local inflammation. 0.1 ml of Triamcinolone acetonide, 5–10 mg/ml, should be injected directly into the lesions and will produce prompt symptom remission. Recurrence, however, is the rule.

Most patients with hidradenitis need definitive surgery. In the most severe cases this means total excision of the axilla or groin skin by an experienced surgeon. Less radical surgery may help if performed by an experienced dermatologist or surgeon. It entails the excision of individual sinus tracts, usually without primary closure or with marsupialization.

HYPERHIDROSIS

Clinical features

Hyperhidrosis is either generalized or local. Generalized hyperhidrosis is usually associated with an internal disorder such as hypothalamic lesions, thyrotoxicosis, fever, lymphomas, phaeochromocytoma and others.

Localized hyperhidrosis is generally restricted to the palms and soles, and/or the axillae. Often related to stress or anxiety, it causes considerable embarrassment and discomfort rather than objective pathology.

Management   Localized hyperhidrosis may be treated with oral anticholinergic drugs but their benefit is limited by the side effects. Applications of 15–25% aluminium chloride in absolute ethanol are usually effective. The solution may be applied at night under polythene occlusion, weekly or monthly according to response. Commercially available aluminium salt preparations help the early stages but there is frequent escape from their sweat-inhibitory effects. Some patients may achieve benefit from counselling to reduce stress and biofeedback. If local treatment fails, iontophoresis or sympathectomy can be considered.

MILIARIASIS

Clinical features   There are two common types of miliaria, miliaria crystallina and miliaria rubra. Miliaria crystallina occurs after sunburn or thermal burns. This occludes the sweat pores, sweating then resulting in small retention vesicles. These are generally asymptomatic and resolve spontaneously or with a mild exfoliating agent such as 3% salicyclic acid in 70% ethanol.

Miliaria rubra (prickly heat) is an erythematous rash of papules and/or vesicles, associated with increased heat, humidity and sweating. The lesions frequently itch or sting. The cause appears to be sweat duct occlusion in the mid or lower epidermis.

Management   The patient should be in a cool, dry environment whenever possible. Soothing, drying lotions such as white shake lotion and the liberal application of zinc stearate powder or talcum powder may help.

FURTHER READING

Fitzpatrick T B et al 1979 Dermatology in general medicine, 2nd edn. McGraw-Hill, New York
Shalita A R et al 1983 Isotretinoin treatment of acne and related disorders: an update. Journal of the American Academy of Dermatology 9: 629–638

R. P. Warin

4. Urticaria

Clinical features Urticaria results when mast cells degranulate to release histamine and other vasoactive mediators. Vasodilation and increased vascular permeability follow causing erythema, oedema and weals, often with severe itching. Angioedema develops when the weal involves subcutaneous tissue. The causes in many cases are never isolated but include allergic, infective, pharmacological and physical reactions.

Acute urticaria lasts a few days whereas chronic urticaria may persist for months or years but its activity often varies. 5% of patients with ordinary chronic urticaria have histologically leucocytoclastic vasculitis. This includes the 1–2% with systemic lupus erythematosus, which should be excluded by tests for anti-nuclear factor and DNA binding.

The differential diagnosis of the cause may be difficult but aids the choice of therapy most likely to be effective. The relative frequency of the different clinical patterns of urticaria in UK hospital practice is shown in Table 4.1.

Table 4.1 Relative frequency of different clinical patterns of urticaria in UK hospital practice

Clinical pattern	Approx. % incidence
Ordinary Urticaria	
Acute	
Chronic (see Fig. 4.1)	72
Angioedema	
Physical Urticaria	
Dermographism (scratch trauma)	10
Cholinergic (exercise, heat) (see Fig. 4.2)	6
Cold	3
Aquagenic direct heat, solar etc	1
Pressure (see Fig. 4.3)	2
Urticarial Vasculitis	5
Hereditary Angioedema (see Fig. 4.4)	1

Management The management of the different types of urticaria can be considered under two main headings, (1) Counselling and general advice and (2) Therapy.

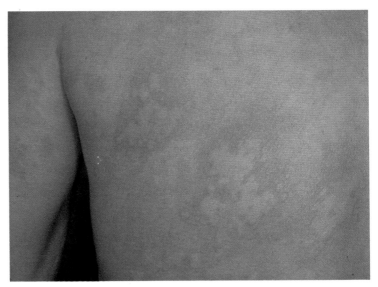

Fig. 4.1 Widespread weals occurring as an aspirin reaction in a patient with chronic urticaria.

Fig. 4.2 Widespread small weals of cholinergic urticaria.

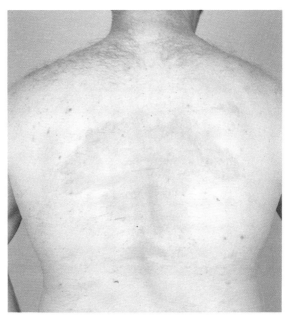

Fig. 4.3 Pressure urticaria 6 hours after pressure against the back of a wooden chair.

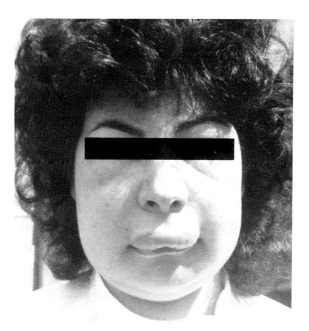

Fig. 4.4 Hereditary angio-oedema. Attack during pregnancy and when off stanozolol.

Counselling and general advice

These are particularly appropriate in the physical urticarias where weals appear in response to particular physical stimuli, e.g. scratch, exercise, heat, cold, water, pressure. The attacks tend to be self-limiting and last 30–60 minutes with the exception of pressure urticaria. Investigations are often unnecessary.

Most patients can be reassured that the condition will settle down over months or years. 'Suggestion' may also play a part, so that a confident plan of action is important. Reassurance and advice over associated psychological stress is often helpful.

Regular exposure to sunlight and 'weather' may reduce the wealing tendency in patients with dermographism and cholinergic urticaria. A threatened attack of cholinergic urticaria may be aborted by rapid cooling. Patients affected by the cold may build up tolerance to cold water by repeated immersion of one limb at a time before the whole body is immersed; this is then continued once or twice a day. It requires patience and stoicism but some have benefited from it.

Various substances can increase the urticarial tendency. In some 30–40% of patients with chronic urticaria, exacerbations will follow salicylates, and in 10–15%, azo dyes and benzoic acid preservatives in foods will have a similar action. It is important to determine whether such exacerbating factors are operating in an individual, as their removal from the diet is often enough to settle the urticaria. This may be done by careful food diary records, elimination diets or test doses of various substances (Challenge Test Battery). The cynic might well point out that the course of chronic urticaria is often 6–9 months and that when the Challenge Test Battery and the dietary control have been completed, the urticaria could be settling spontaneously. Undoubtedly, in chronic urticaria, patience, time and care by the physician is often rewarding.

Autohaemotherapy and calcium injections have been popular measures against chronic urticaria in the past. Rightly or wrongly, they are rarely used nowadays.

If all seems lost, a complete change of environment or admission to hospital sometimes leads to remission.

Therapy

Antihistamines. Antihistamines remain the mainstay of treatment. Histamine Type I receptor blockers (H_1-blockers) reduce the size of the weal and itching and their regular daily use gives considerable relief, particularly in severe cases. Formerly the art of treatment was to give a particular antihistamine in a dose and at a time to reduce or suppress weals without troublesome side-effects. As many patients are active young adults, the newer antihistamines without sedative side-effects— terfenadine 60 mg twice daily or possibly astemizole 10 mg once a day— have been of great value, as symptoms can be more readily relieved without limiting the patients' activities.

If a histamine Type II receptor blocker (H_2-blocker) such as cimetidine or ranitidine is added to the H_1-blocker the effect on the weals is increased. However, the same effect can often be obtained by raising the dose of the H_1-blocker. At best they are only likely to give slight help.

Antihistamines can be given regularly or intermittently to cover periods of likely exposure to precipitating factors, such as a few hours before an expected cold exposure in a patient with cold urticaria. Of the older antihistamines, cyproheptadine is said to have more effect in cold urticaria. Antihistamines are not effective in pressure urticaria except when there is coincidental chronic urticaria.

Corticosteroids.   Corticosteroids may reduce the wealing tendency but only with adequate doses. Except for the temporary control of severe phases, the use of corticosteroids in chronic urticaria is contraindicated. Where treatment is needed for pressure urticaria systemic corticosteroids may help but large doses may be required. In some patients, prednisone for 1–2 days after any activity likely to produce pressure-induced weals will help to reduce their severity. Corticosteroids are also the most effective treatment for urticarial vasculitis in large adequate doses and for prolonged periods. However, in many cases the condition will gradually settle without resorting to them. They should be reserved for patients with very severe persistent urticaria or with complications.

Small doses of anabolic steroids have successfully reduced the frequency and severity of attacks of hereditary angioedema. Stanazolol 2.5–10 mg daily, and danazol 100–400 mg daily have been given regularly for long periods. The correct dose is the smallest to give clinical relief. Care is required in children as puberty could be slightly delayed.

As with other indications, patients who have been treated with systemic corticosteroids for long periods or at high doses may have adrenocortical suppression and appropriate precautions need to be taken.

C1—esterase inhibitor sparing agents   Patients with hereditary angioedema (autosomal dominant transmission) go through phases of swellings, sometimes initiated by trauma or general physical tiredness. Tranexamic acid (1–1.5 g, two to three times a day) spares the C1 esterase inhibitor and regular treatment undoubtedly helps to reduce the frequency and severity of attacks.

FURTHER READING

Warin R P, Champion R H 1974, Urticaria. Saunders, Lloyd-Luke

T. W. Stewart

5. Cutaneous Tumours

Skin tumours occur at any age. However, they are unusual in children except for the common wart of viral origin and molluscum contagiosum papules, both of which are discussed in Chapter 1.

WARTY OR EPIDERMAL NAEVI

Clinical features Warty or epidermal naevi (Fig. 5.1) are most commonly seen on the face and neck at the sites of embryonic clefts. They are almost always present from birth and may extend well down a limb. Small areas may be difficult to distinguish from viral warts but some contain sebaceous glands or other skin appendages and may have a yellow tint.

Management This should be by surgical shaving or excision and is best done by a plastic surgeon.

PYOGENIC GRANULOMA

Clinical features Pyogenic granuloma (Fig. 5.2) is one of the great misnomers in dermatology since it is neither pyogenic in origin nor a granuloma. It is an acutely arising capillary haemangioma which grows rapidly, distends and then usually ruptures the overlying skin. This leaves a naked mass of delicate blood vessels which tear and bleed copiously with the most minimal trauma. They can arise anywhere on the body and at any age and because of the bleeding they can constitute that rarity of rarities, a dermatological emergency.

Management This is by curettage and cauterization under local anaesthetic. When occasionally they recur, the same therapy may be needed again.

SKIN TAGS

Clinical features Skin tags (Fig. 5.3) are very common, especially in women and particularly in brunettes. They occur mainly around the neck and in the

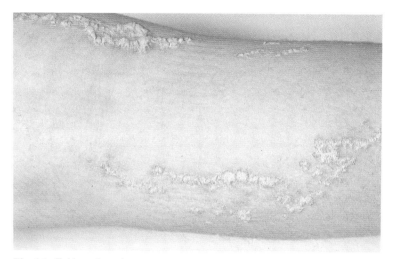

Fig. 5.1   Epidermal naevi.

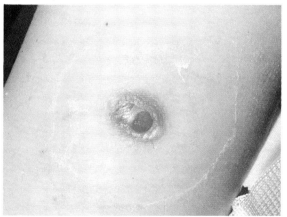

Fig. 5.2   Pyogenic granuloma.

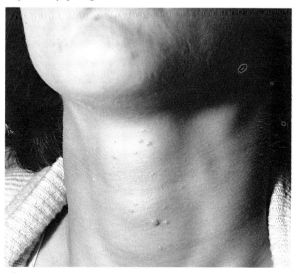

Fig. 5.3   Skin tags.

axillae but can be found anywhere on the body; although usually tiny they occasionally become as large as a hazelnut. Often misdiagnosed as warts, they are merely floppy excrescences of epidermis with a fibrovascular core. Some contain naevus cells and are therefore really filiform moles.

Management   This is to cut through the pedicle with a cautery under local anaesthesia.

DERMATOFIBROMA

Clinical features   The dermatofibroma (Fig. 5.4) is most common on the exposed parts of the limbs of women, although it can occur on any part of the body and is also found in men. A fibrous nodule, looking and feeling like a lentil in the skin, it is usually some 5 mm in diameter and is thought to result from previous minor injury, especially insect bites. Early lesions are softer and contain histiocytes, hence the alternative name of histiocytoma. Some are very vascular and rupture of the tiny vessels results in haemosiderin deposition and hence pigmentation. This type is sometimes called a sclerosing angioma.

Management   This is by excision under local anaesthesia.

CORNS

Clinical features   Corns (Fig. 5.5) are very common tumours of the feet, mainly on and around the toes. They are due to pressure which squeezes the skin on to the underlying bones causing the epidermis to produce a hyperkeratotic layer as a protection from erosion.

Management   Management of corns is, therefore, a problem for the orthopaedic surgeon and all that can be done medically is to soften the lesion with keratolytics such as 10% salicylic acid in yellow soft paraffin; however, this treatment is merely palliative. Soft corns can occur in the toe clefts—usually the fourth. The simplest treatment is to separate the toes with a rubber wedge but, in addition, the application of 10% salicylic acid in industrial methylated spirits as a daily paint with daily paring down speeds their resolution.

SEBORRHOEIC WARTS

Clinical features   The seborrhoeic wart or seborrhoeic keratosis (Fig. 5.6) occurs anywhere on almost everybody's skin after the age of 40 years or so. It starts as a pale yellow or brownish papule with a slightly greasy 'feel'. With time it often becomes dark or even black, with a warty, sometimes dimpled surface. It appears to be stuck on to the skin rather than arising in it, but

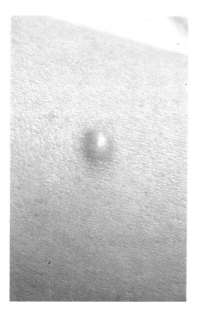

Fig. 5.4 Dermatofibroma.

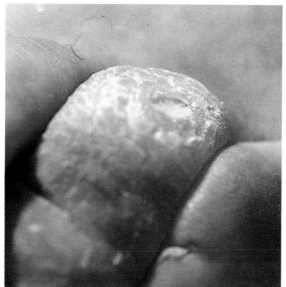

Fig. 5.5 Corns.

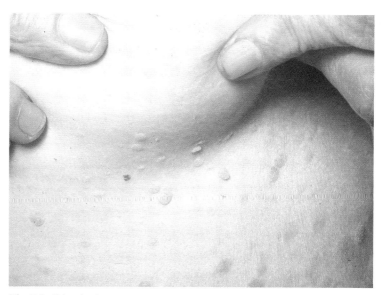

Fig. 5.6 Seborrhoeic warts.

occasionally seborrhoeic warts can be pedunculated. They never become malignant so they are removed only for cosmetic reasons or because they catch on clothing. Rarely, seborrhoeic warts erupt with large numbers appearing in the course of a few weeks. This phenomenon, the so-called Leser-Trélat sign, can be associated with an internal malignancy, usually of the gastrointestinal tract.

Management   Management of seborrhoeic warts is removal by curettage under local anaesthesia or by cryotherapy.

SQUAMOUS PAPILLOMA

Clinical features The squamous papilloma (Fig. 5.7) is a wart-like nodule usually on the face of an elderly person.

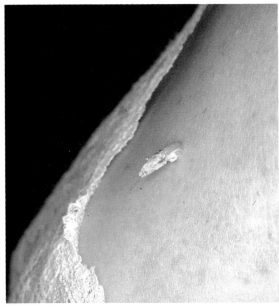

Fig. 5.7 Squamous papilloma.

Management Curettage and cauterization under local anaesthesia or by cryotherapy is the treatment of choice.

EPIDERMOID CYSTS

Clinical features The most common cystic tumour is probably the sebaceous cyst (Fig. 5.8), better called an epidermoid cyst. Occurring anywhere on the body, it is a firm, slightly soft swelling with a central punctum. The cheesy material it contains is keratin, not sebum.

Management The treatment of choice is excision. A similar swelling (but without a central punctum) occurs usually on the scalp. This is technically a pilar cyst, being derived from a particular part of a hair follicle; treatment is also by excision.

MILIA

Clinical features Milia (Fig. 5.9) are pinhead-sized glistening white epidermoid cysts most commonly seen on the upper cheeks and around the eyes in young adults, especially females. They arise in undeveloped sebaceous glands and they often appear after sunbathing.

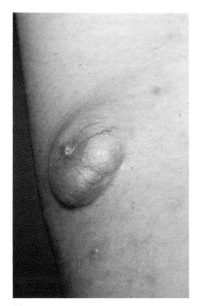

Fig. 5.8 Epidermoid cyst.

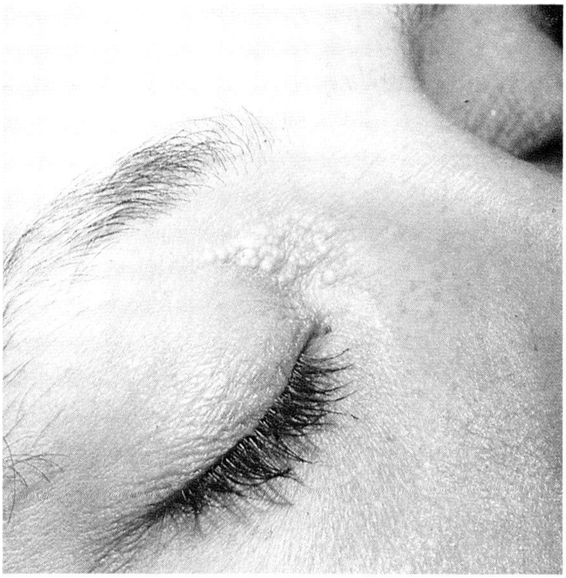

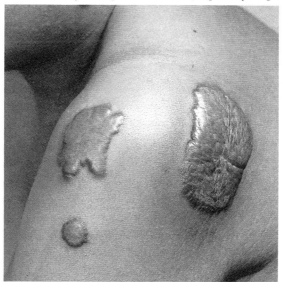

Fig. 5.9 Milia.

Management Management is to incise them and express the contents with the round side of a curette end or to lift them out with a pointed scalpel blade or a sterile hypodermic needle. Milia are occasionally seen elsewhere after sub-epidermal blistering such as is caused by second-degree burns, bullous pemphigoid and epidermolysis bullosa.

KELOIDS

Clinical features Keloids (Fig. 5.10) arise from excessive production of collagen in the dermis, usually in response to trauma, especially surgical or that caused

Fig. 5.10 Keloids.

by burns. Negroes are particularly prone to produce keloids after injury and this should be borne in mind when contemplating surgery on them.

Management   The treatment of choice is by intralesional steroid injections which use the known catabolic effect of steroids on collagen, especially that which has been recently formed. Keloids should not be excised because experience has shown that if a patient has a tendency to form keloids, another keloid appears following surgery. The pre-sternal area is particularly prone to produce keloids following injury or inflammation, particularly that associated with acne vulgaris.

MOLES OR MELANOCYTIC NAEVI

Clinical features   Moles or melanocytic naevi (Fig. 5.11) occur on every normal skin irrespective of its colour and are usually important for cosmetic reasons only. They are common in childhood and young adult life and most adults have from 10–20 pigmented moles. They may be brown or black macules caused by an increase in melanocytes at the dermo-epidermal junction but, as they age, the pigment cells drop down into the dermis and produce compound naevi, which may be skin coloured or brown and may have hairs growing from them. An eruption of moles can occur in both sexes at puberty and also in pregnancy.

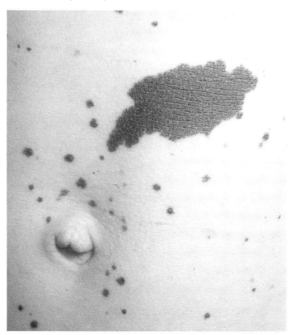

Fig. 5.11 Moles.

Management   This is by excision or cautery, mostly for cosmetic reasons but infants born with extensive deeply pigmented hairy naevi should have them removed and grafted as they carry an increased risk of malignancy.

BASAL-CELL CARCINOMA

Clinical features

The basal-cell carcinoma (basal-cell epithelioma or rodent ulcer) (Fig. 5.12) is usually on the face or neck, nearly always after the age of 50 years. However, it can arise anywhere and in young people. The early lesion is a small, smooth papule which over several months or years enlarges to a rounded lesion with pearly nodules in a rolled edge, over which small dilated blood vessels course. There is sometimes a central ulcer which may crust and this needs to be removed with a pair of forceps for the characteristic pearly edge to be seen. However, not all basal-cell epitheliomata ulcerate and some histologically cystic lesions often remain solid. In some, a fibrous reaction produces a sclerodermatous appearance; marked pigmentation may sometimes occur, leading to a suspicion that the lesion is a malignant melanoma.

The basal-cell carcinoma only very rarely metastasizes but it can be very destructive locally, even penetrating bone such as the skull, in which case death may result from sepsis. If the patient complains of a chronic crusted ulcer on the face, particularly after trauma while shaving in a man, or a slight scratch on the face in a woman, a basal-cell epithelioma should be suspected. The minor trauma only draws attention to the early lesion; it has no aetiological role.

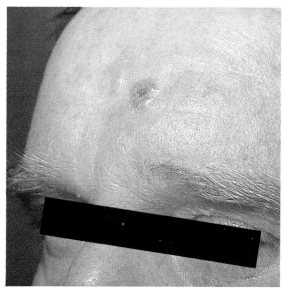

Fig. 5.12 Basal-cell carcinoma.

Management

As with any skin tumour, if the diagnosis is uncertain a biopsy should be carried out; this may be purely diagnostic or an excision biopsy. The best treatment of a basal-cell carcinoma is surgery, preferably by a plastic surgeon if the cosmetic appearance is important. An excellent end result can be achieved and the availability of the surgical specimen means that histological examination can show whether the tumour has been completely removed. Sometimes in the elderly and infirm, curettage and cauterization may be the kindest treatment despite the relatively high recurrence rate. Cryotherapy with liquid nitrogen is effective and 5% 5-fluorouracil cream can be tried in superficial basal-cell carcinomata.

X-irradiation with fractionation techniques is less commonly used than it was: the resultant necrotic ulcer heals with an avascular scar which readily breaks down, even years later, and becomes infected (radionecrosis). The scar is often unsightly and the absence of a surgical specimen means that there is no certainty that the tumour has been completely destroyed. The use of X-rays over cartilage and around the orbit and nose can also be technically difficult.

KERATO-ACANTHOMA

Clinical features

The kerato-acanthoma (Fig. 5.13) is pathogenetically on the borderline between hyperplasia and neoplasia. It is found mainly on the face and backs of the hands, grows rapidly for about 2 months, often reaching 1–2 cm in diamater. It remains static for a further 2 months, then over a similar period involutes leaving a somewhat unsightly pitted scar. At its maximum, it is a dome-shaped yellowish nodule with a rounded edge across which blood vessels course, and a central keratinous plug which, if removed, reveals more keratin; this helps to distinguish a kerato-acanthoma from a basal-cell epithelioma. The speed of growth is very much more rapid than that of a squamous-cell carcinoma.

Management

Treatment of choice is curettage in one piece with cauterization of the base under local anaesthesia. This removes the lesion, gives a better scar and allows histological examination. This is important because occasionally a lesion which clinically and histologically appears to be a kerato-acanthoma later behaves like a squamous-cell carcinoma.

SOLAR KERATOSES

Clinical features

Solar, actinic or senile keratoses (Fig. 5.14) arise, as the name suggests, on skin exposed to sunshine for a lengthy period—the more intense the sunshine and the paler the skin, the shorter the necessary exposure. The lesions are superficial scaly roughenings of the skin often more easily felt than seen. Mainly on the face, bald scalp and the backs of the hands and wrists, they may, if left alone, progress to form squamous-cell carcinomata but only a small percentage actually undergo this change.

Management

Cauterization, excision, cryotherapy or, if there are many, 5% 5-fluorouracil cream may be applied twice daily to the lesions after a preliminary wash with soap and water. The antimitotic drug is absorbed by the dysplastic cells which are promptly destroyed. The patient must be warned that the skin will become angry and sore but treatment must continue for 6 weeks. Once therapy is complete, an antibiotic cream may be needed for any secondary sepsis. The result is always excellent since there should be no scar.

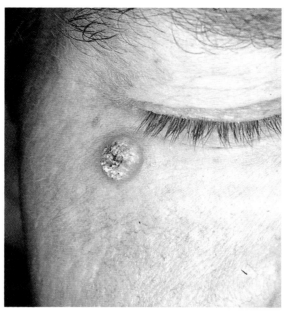

Fig. 5.13   Kerato-acanthoma.

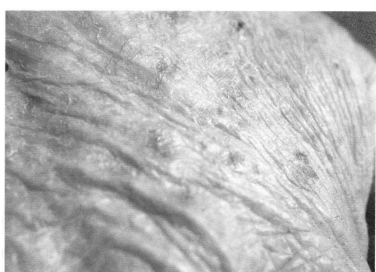

Fig. 5.14   Solar keratosis.

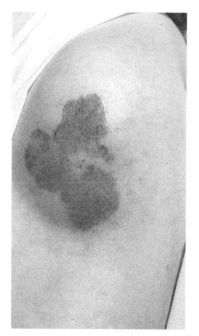

Fig. 5.15   Bowen's disease of the skin.

BOWEN'S DISEASE OF THE SKIN

Clinical features   Bowen's disease of the skin (intra-epidermal carcinoma or carcinoma-in-situ of the skin) (Fig. 5.15) is becoming increasingly common. It develops in people over 50 years of age and can resemble a patch of psoriasis or eczema anywhere on the body. It is usually present for several years before the steadily enlarging, scaly, non-itching plaque arouses suspicion of something other than a benign skin reaction. The edge is irregular but well-defined; quite large areas can become involved but change into frank invasive squamous-cell carcinoma is unusual. Biopsy may be needed to confirm the diagnosis.

Management Treatment is preferably by excision. Curettage, cryotherapy, X-irradiation and the use of 5% 5-fluorouracil cream are all useful.

SQUAMOUS-CELL CARCINOMA

Clinical features A squamous-cell carcinoma is usually a nodule (Fig. 5.16) which grows quite quickly (but not as quickly as a kerato-acanthoma). An eroded, heaped-up cauliflower lesion results, commonly on exposed sites if sunshine is the main cause but, if there is an occupational element, the lesion can appear on covered skin. An example is the scrotum of an engineering worker. Instead of appearing as a lump, it may present as an ulcer with everted edges. Areas of persistent inflammation, such as patches of chronic discoid lupus erythematosus or lupus vulgaris, may become the site of a squamous-cell carcinoma.

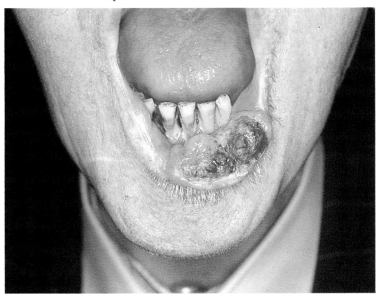

Fig. 5.16 Squamous-cell carcinoma.

Management This is by surgery or radiotherapy or both, if necessary, and a watch should be kept for the metastases which some lesions may produce.

MALIGNANT MELANOMA

Clinical features Malignant melanoma (Fig. 5.17) is increasing in many parts of the world. Some 25% are thought to arise from existing moles but most develop de

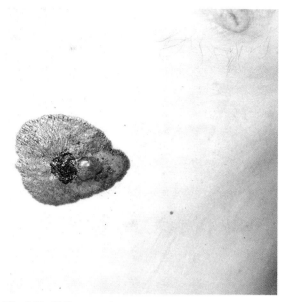

Fig. 5.17   Malignant melanoma.

novo, and from such sites as the choroid in the eye and the substantia
nigra in the central nervous system. There is an increased incidence of
malignant melanoma in white skins in sunny climates but it appears that
the risk of a mole becoming malignant is of the order of one in a million.

Management   If a mole shows increasing depth of pigmentation, spillage of pigment
into the surrounding skin, increase in size, crusting or bleeding, an
excision biopsy is mandatory and this is best done by a plastic surgeon. It
is important to appreciate that although 'messing about with moles
makes them malignant' is a myth, changes in a mole mean that its
removal is essential, together with any clinically involved lymph nodes.
Radiotherapy and chemotherapy are usually of little assistance.

SECONDARY DEPOSITS

Clinical features   Primary carcinomas of internal organs, especially the bronchus and
breast, may produce secondary deposits in the skin (Fig. 5.18).
Occasionally tumours of other organs and blood dyscrasias are
responsible. The lesions are usually reddish-brown, single or multiple,
painless, hard nodules in the dermis. The diagnosis is confirmed by
biopsy.

Management   Management is essentially that of the primary lesion.

BIOPSY

If the nature of any tumour is not obvious, a biopsy, easily and quickly
done under local anaesthesia, is essential. The histology of a small but

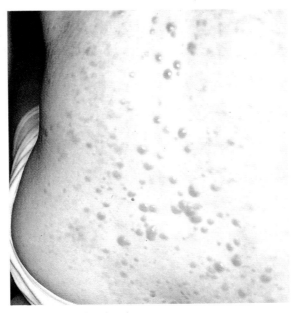

Fig. 5.18 Secondary deposits.

representative portion of the tumour should give a clear diagnosis and
the appropriate treatment can be instituted.

SURGICAL TECHNIQUES

Cryotherapy

In this procedure, tissue is destroyed by freezing, using either solid
carbon dioxide (CO_2 snow), CO_2 slush or liquid nitrogen. CO_2 snow is
produced by allowing the gas from a cylinder to expand into a chamois
leather bag held tightly over the open orifice of the cylinder.
Alternatively, a small apparatus is available utilising bulb-sized cylinders,
the gas expanding into a small chamber from which it can be pushed into
a tube, emerging as a solid stick.

Freezing with solid CO_2 is relatively slow (requiring $2-3$ minutes of
application) and a quicker effect is obtained using a slush made by
placing the CO_2 snow in a galley-pot and adding a few drops of acetone:
application for a few seconds will be all that is needed. Liquid nitrogen
requires a Dewar flask for transport but because of the lower
temperatures reached, it is more effective than either solid CO_2 or
CO_2 slush. It is dabbed on to the lesion using a cotton wool pledget or
used in a special apparatus either to produce a jet or to cool a cryoprobe.

Diathermy

This technique employs electrical current to produce intense heat. If a
monoterminal current is used, the needle is inserted into the lesion

(electrodessication) or a spark can be created between the needle and the lesion (fulguration). Alternatively, a twin-terminal holder can be employed, the tissue damage being produced by a spark between the terminals.

Electrolysis is a variation of electrodessication used for the destruction of hair follicles. The needle is inserted down a follicle to destroy the hair. It remains mainly a cosmetic procedure for hirsutes and may be used in the treatment of small vascular lesions.

Cauterization

The cautery uses an electric current to heat up a platinum tip which is made in a variety of shapes for differing purposes. The method can be used on its own or, because of the effective haemostasis produced, after curettage.

Curettage

This means destruction or eradication of a lesion by means of a small spoon, the edge of which is very sharp. It is usually followed by electrocautery.

Biopsy

An elliptical piece of tissue is excised to be submitted for histological examination, to try to make a diagnosis on mystifying lesions. Usually a specimen approximately 10 mm long, 2 mm wide and 2 mm deep and crossing the boundary between normal and abnormal skin will suffice. It should preferably be handled using a skin hook rather than forceps and placed in a specimen bottle containing formalin-saline or rapidly frozen if immunofluorescence studies are indicated. The wound always requires careful suturing to try to obtain a good cosmetic result. Occasionally, a punch biopsy can be taken using an instrument rather like a cork-borer. This technique is often used for research purposes but very small lesions can be removed this way. Suturing is not usually necessary.

Excision

The technique is the same as that described for the biopsy but because the amount of tissue being removed is usually greater, care must be especially directed to the lines of incision, haemostasis and suturing in order to minimise scarring. Occasionally, instead of excising a benign lesion it may be shaved flat, level with the surrounding area of skin: if necessary, cautery or cryotherapy may follow this procedure.

Local anaesthetic technique

With the exception of cryotherapy, all these techniques require local anaesthesia. To induce local anaesthesia a dental syringe is used, which holds cartridges containing 1–2% lignocaine. Use fine, flexible needles. Adrenaline may be added to reduce bleeding especially on the face and scalp but it should be used with care or avoided altogether on digits and the end of the nose.

FURTHER READING

A J Rook, D S Wilkinson, F J Ebling (eds) 1979 Textbook of Dermatology, 3rd edn. Blackwell Scientific Publications, Oxford, p 2129–2232

V. Cassis

6. Leg Ulcers

Leg ulcers may present diagnostic and therapeutic problems. There are three main types:
1. Venous ulcers
2. Arterial ulcers
3. Vasculitis alone or in any combination
A combination of any of the three also occurs. Their prevalence has recently been described by Gilmore and Wheeland (1982).

VENOUS (stasis) ULCERS

Clinical features Chronically raised venous pressure in the lower limbs results in oedema, purpura, eczema and pigmentation, and may progress to stasis ulceration. It is the most common type of leg ulcer in adults. It can appear at any age after puberty but most often between 40 and 70 years. The treatment period is often prolonged. Relapse is more frequent in the elderly. Patients may have aching discomfort in the limb, nocturnal muscle cramps and pain relieved by rest and elevation of the leg.

Such ulcers (Fig. 6.1) usually occur near the malleoli, where the skin is oedematous, eczematous and pigmented. The oedema results in poorer tissue oxygenation so that the skin becomes less resistant to endogenous and exogenous stimuli. The area overlying the malleolus, especially the medial, is the commonest site of ulceration.

Stasis ulcers may be of any size. The base is usually moist with extensive granulations and secondary infection is common. The surrounding skin temperature is normal, the arterial pulses are palpable and varicose veins are present. Clinical tests such as Trendelenburg's and Perthes' demonstrate venous reflux and the state of competence of the deep venous system.

Management Causes of bilateral peripheral oedema, e.g. cardiac or renal disease, should be looked for and treated if necessary. Diuretics may be helpful.

Iron deficiency anaemia commonly coexists and must be corrected. The significance of low plasma zinc levels is unclear but some patients may benefit from oral zinc sulphate therapy (220 mg twice daily).

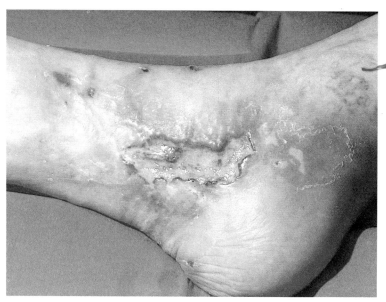

Fig. 6.1 A venous ulcer.

Medicated bandages such as zinc paste and ichthammol bandage or zinc paste, calamine and clioquinol bandage are useful (Fig. 6.2). To increase the efficiency of the leg muscle pump and thus increase venous return, elastic bandaging is the single essential part of treatment (Fig. 6.3). Elevation also helps. Some patients become sensitized to rubber in elastic bandages. Alternatives are available but expensive.

Patients with gravitational disease often have their problems compounded by the unwise use of sensitizers such as neomycin,

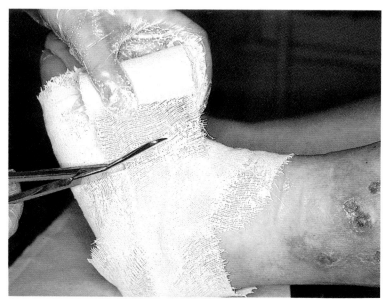

Fig. 6.2 Bandaging technique. Application of medicated bandage.

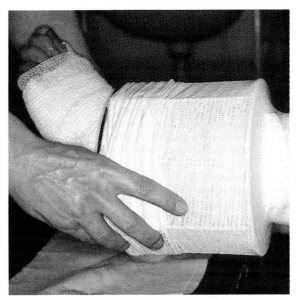

Fig. 6.3 Bandaging technique. Application of tubigrip.

framycetin, soframycin, sulphonamides, antihistamines, mercurial salts and clioquinol. Lanolin and preservatives in local preparations may also sensitise.

Weeping ulcers and *acute dermatitis* are best treated initially by wet compresses of 0.02% potassium permanganate, 0.1% silver nitrate, 0.8% aluminium acetate, 0.25−0.5% chloramine or 0.9% saline which should be changed every 5−6 hours. Subsequently, ulcers should be given a drying application of carbowax, 1500 with 0.2 or 1.0% chlorhexidine, 10−20% propylene glycol or 0.8% aluminium acetate or proteolytic enzymes, and eczema a mild corticosteroid cream once or twice a day. A solution of 1% eosin may be applied once a day to small wet skin defects.

Pathogens are often found in ulcers, resulting in secondary infection in the lesions. Beta-haemolytic streptococci should always be treated seriously, usually by systemic penicillin. Ulcers secondarily infected by a synergistic combination of *Staphylococcus aureus* and streptococci should be treated with systemic antibiotics.

Applications to dry ulcers may be ointments of 0.25% silver nitrate, 0.2−1.0% chlorhexidine or a dextranomer powder.

Chronic eczema with dry, scaly, red skin around an ulcer should be treated with ointments or pastes containing zinc oxide with sulphur, tar or salicylic acid, or with a mild corticosteroid ointment if itchy. Paste bandages may break the itch/scratch vicious cycle. Some very painful ulcers, resistant to topical treatments, may become less painful and heal quickly under an hydrocolloid occlusive dressing such as Geliperm or Surgicare® . It should be changed only once or twice a week. No cutaneous hypersensitivity has yet been observed from these dressings. Some leg ulcers are refractory to conservative treatment. Skin grafting may cover the ulcer and relieve pains. Split-skin grafts or pinch grafts of autologous skin are taken under local anaesthesia.

ARTERIAL ULCERS

Clinical features Several organic arterial diseases lower capillary blood flow in the legs resulting in ischaemia and ulceration. Arteriosclerosis is the commonest. Patients have severe pain, which is relieved by hanging their feet down over the edge of the bed. They complain of coldness and hypoaesthesia of the feet. The skin is usually cold, atrophic, hairless and dry, and nail growth is often impeded. Severe skin ischaemia results in ulceration which usually starts at the tip of the toes, on the heel and achilles region as a dark pustule which ulcerates and is surrounded by a zone of cyanosis. They tend to be multiple, punched-out and shallow (Fig. 6.4). Elevating the leg quickly produces pallor: it becomes bright red and the veins fill slowly when dependent. The pulses are absent or reduced which can be verified by oscillometry and Doppler testing. Distal blood pressure measurement and angiography may be needed to delineate the extent of the disease.

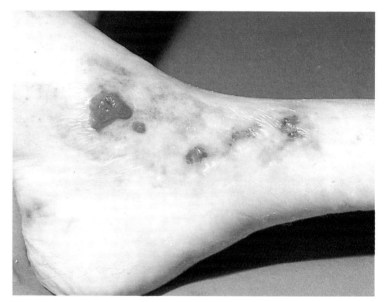

Fig. 6.4 An arterial ulcer.

Management Bed rest with appropriate physiotherapy is important. Smoking must be prohibited. Vasodilator and platelet anti-aggregating drugs, e.g. aspirin, may improve peripheral circulation and thus healing. Mild sedatives may also reduce vasomotor tone. Compressive bandaging is contraindicated and anaemia and heart failure must be corrected. Sometimes if the distal blood pressure is reasonably high (> 20 mm Hg), complete excision of an ulcer and its surrounding rim of infarcted tissue, followed by a split-skin graft to the deep fascia may be successful. Some ulcers do not heal on conservative therapy. Sympathectomy and/or arterial bypass surgery may be needed if the arterial block is above the knee. Amputation is frequently the end result of lower limb arterial ulceration.

VASCULITIS

Clinical features   The site of pathology in vasculitis may be capillaries, venules and arteries, alone or in any combination. Often it is the cutaneous sign of complex pathology initiated by, for example, infections, drug allergy or autoimmune disease. The onset is often abrupt, with itching, burning or stinging. Some patients show various reactions, including necrotic ulcers. The lesions are skin micro-infarctions usually bilateral and symmetrical on the legs.

Management   A thorough history and physical examination, specific laboratory tests and skin histology, including immunofluorescent studies, should be done as soon as possible to establish the cause. The presence of cardiac, hepatic or renal failure, arterial hypertension, anaemia, malnutrition or other serious general disease must be sought. The domestic conditions and social and occupational background must be assessed.

Correct therapy depends on recognising the underlying cause of vasculitic leg ulcers; it may be drug withdrawal, antibiotics, corticosteroids, or bed rest. Simple local treatment such as that for gravitational disease must be started. The long-term results of therapy vary.

Adhesive hydrocolloid occlusive dressings, suitable for the different types of leg ulcer, offer convenience and cost-effective treatment. Early surgical intervention for varices, skin-grafting and arterial by-pass may promote healing, save potentially dangerous, costly and prolonged bed rest and give patients a more pleasant life.

FURTHER READING

Gilmore W A, Wheeland R G 1982 Treatment of ulcers on legs by pinch grafts and a supportive dressing of polyurethane. Journal of Dermatologic Surgery and Oncology 8: 177

Roenigk H H, Young J R 1975 Leg Ulcers. Harper & Row, Hagerstown, Maryland

Verdich J, Anderson B L 1980 Leg ulcers. A retrospective investigation of a ten-year hospital material. Ugeskrift for Laeger 142: 3248

C. F. H. Vickers

7. Endogenous Eczema

This chapter is concerned with endogenous eczema, of which there are four prime types:
1. Atopic eczema
2. Seborrhoeic eczema
3. Discoid eczema
4. Pompholyx

Clinical features   Eczema is characterised by the presence of erythema and small vesicle formation which may be multi-locular on palms and soles. Lichenification may occur (Fig. 7.1) and often there is evidence of scratching. The disease is pruritic.

Atopic eczema is a specific, immunologically-determined disorder often

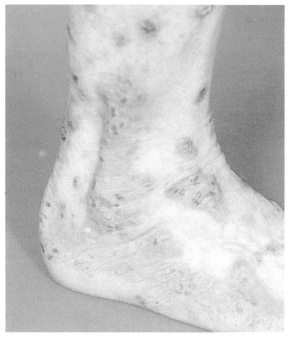

Fig. 7.1 Lichenification.

associated with asthma, hay fever and ichthyosis. It affects between 5 and 20% of the population, with a higher incidence in the Western world. The diagnosis is made by the classical distribution of the lesions usually on the face, antecubital and popliteal fossae in children; on the face, neck and antecubital fossae in adults. The vast majority (85–90%) of children with infantile eczema clear spontaneously during childhood. Adverse prognostic features are late-onset (after 2 years) and involvement of the knees and elbows. The disease in childhood is distressing to patient and family and its favourable natural history should not result in a failure to use effective therapy. These children have a low resistance to herpes simplex and other viruses (see Ch. 1).

Seborrhoeic eczema, a misnomer as sebaceous glands are not involved in the disorder, is a pattern of endogenous eczema which usually consists of otitis externa, blepharitis, naso-labial fold eczema, dandruff and flexural eczema with involvement of the shield area of the chest and back.

Discoid eczema (nummular eczema) usually occurs in people over 60 but can occur at any age and is characterised by discoid or coin-shaped lesions usually scattered on the limbs.

Pompholyx has to be separated, though it is only a special name for eczema affecting the palms and soles. Because of the anatomical site, the veiscles become larger, multi-locular and remain intact for longer periods thus requiring somewhat different specific treatment.

Management

General measures

These apply to all forms of eczema. Avoiding local heat and contact with irritants such as soap and detergents are of prime importance. If secondary infection is present or suspected, a course of systemic antibiotics is indicated. Many believe that all eczematous patients are secondarily invaded by microbes and that systemic antibiotics may reduce the severity of the disease.

Patients with any type of eczema should be discouraged from working in an occupation such as the engineering industry, where contact with coolant oil may aggravate it or the building industry where contact with cement and sand may have an irritant and then sensitizing potential. Patients with widespread eczema often find comfort by wearing cotton pyjamas under daytime clothing. This has a two-fold purpose of preventing the staining of clothing and a soothing effect.

Atopic eczema

Local therapy. The general principles of therapy have been outlined; local therapy in this condition is three-fold. Topical corticosteroids are extremely important and will usually contain the disease. The weakest possible corticosteroids should be used for routine maintenance but in acute exacerbations high potency topical corticosteroids may be applied for a few days, with a slow return to a low potency steriod. This should be done by either using more dilute steroids, preferably in the pharmaceutically-produced dilutions or step-wise down through a series of topical corticosteroids. It is always important to monitor risk/benefit ratios. A minor degree of steroid atrophy may be acceptable in a patient with otherwise uncontrollable pruritus but this should always be discussed with the patient. Stunting of growth in atopic children treated with topical steroids has been a subject of argument for some years but most believe that the stunting is a result of the disease rather than the use of topical corticosteroids.

The second line of attack is emollients. Most patients have xerosis or ichthyosis vulgaris. Adding an emollient to the regime considerably reduces the consumption of topical corticosteroids and is more comfortable for the patient. Emulsifying ointment or aqueous cream may be used after a bath at night or an emollient bath oil may be used. It has been suggested that emollients alone plus ultra-violet light will control some atopic childhood eczema.

Tar-containing preparations are the third element of local treatment. Crude coal tar is the most effective, applied usually in Lassar's paste, though it may be used in other bases. In tropical and humid climates it should be very carefully considered as it often induces miliariasis and folliculitis. Occlusive bandaging with tar, hydroxyquinolone or ichthyol-containing bandages is very helpful, especially in children with atopic eczema. This, too, is sometimes difficult in humid tropical climates.

Systemic therapy.   The use of systemic antihistamines with soporific side effects such as promethazine and trimeprazine is probably the pivotal point in the management of the atopic infant and young child. Large doses are required as these drugs appear to be metabolised more rapidly by infants and children than by adults. More modern antihistamines with little or no soporific side effects are valueless in their management. Systemic corticosteroids or adrenocorticotrophic hormone (ACTH) are never justified in childhood or infancy but may be required in adults. For them, ACTH or long-acting tetracosactrin are probably the most useful drugs given at weekly or fortnightly intervals with gradual dose reduction. (See Ch. 22 for systemic therapy with other drugs and for dietary factors.)

Seborrhoeic eczema   This is frequently complicated by staphylococcal or candidal superinfection. Thus, giving systemic antibiotics in acute exacerbations is often very helpful and topical antibiotic/corticosteroid preparations are mandatory. Local tar should never be applied to these patients. Although there is no scientific rationale for it, sulphur and ichthyol-containing preparations often help.

Discoid eczema   Management is very similar to that of atopic eczema with greater emphasis on the use of tar-containing preparations. Secondary infection is frequent and a steroid antibiotic combination should be added to the regime.

Pompholyx   Cheiro pompholyx and pedo pompholyx are respectively eczema of the palms (Fig. 7.2) and soles. They commonly present with large, intact bullae which should be ruptured under clean conditions, followed by soaking in tepid 1/10 000 potassium permanganate solution and wet

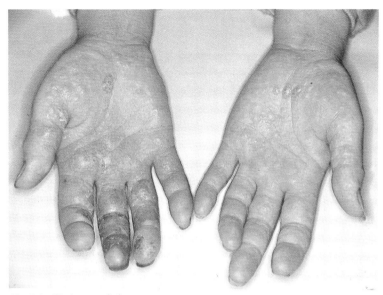

Fig. 7.2   Cheiro pompholyx.

dressings of 0.5% silver nitrate, normal saline or Burows solution which are both soothing and effective. Topical corticosteroids are valueless in the acute phase but systemic antibiotics are often indicated for the frequent secondary infection, particularly on the soles.

In contact allergic eczema, management is the recognition of the allergen and, if possible, its removal from the patient's environment. Spontaneous resolution usually follows but short-term topical corticosteroid therapy may be needed to relieve symptoms and shorten the duration of the disease.

Many patients with hand and foot eczema develop severe hyperkeratosis. Salicyclic acid 5–20% in white soft paraffin prevents fissuring and thus potential secondary infection.

FURTHER READING

Rajka G 1975 Atopic dermatitis. W B Saunders, Lloyd Luke, Philadelphia
Wilkinson D A 1977 Nursing and management of skin disease: a guide to practical dermatology for doctors and nurses. Faber, London

R. E. Church

8. Contact and Industrial Dermatoses

INTRODUCTION

In this chapter dermatitis signifies contact dermatitis and eczema signifies endogenous eczema.

Dermatitis may be an allergic or irritant response. The commonest occupational skin disease, it always starts at the point of maximum contact with the irritant or sensitizer, usually the hands. However, almost anything in the general environment has at some time been incriminated as a skin irritant. Prevention is most important in dermatitis management but, once established, the identification and removal of the cause is vital.

INVESTIGATION

A thorough history is the most important pointer to the cause of dermatitis.

When?

When did it start and have there been previous attacks? If so was the subject in the same occupation? Is it worse at work and does it improve at weekends or during holidays? Is it seasonal? Traumatic dermatitis tends to be worse in cold weather. A seasonal history might also point to plants or sunlight as the cause.

Where?

Dermatitis begins at the point of maximum contact of the irritant or sensitizer. It is therefore common on the hands, but if the eyelids are first affected, this suggests sensitivity either to a vapour or dust. Starting on covered areas it is more likely to be due to clothes, though accumulation of dust, as in coal miners, can cause frictional dermatitis (where the clothing rubs). The spread is also instructive; severe dermatitis of the hands may give rise to an eruption on the feet which is usually mild. If the eruption starts on the feet and then attacks the hands, it is more likely to be due to shoe dermatitis or tinea pedis than to an industrial contact.

Occupation

A detailed description of the patient's occupation is required, including the materials which he handles, recent changes and the protective clothing worn. If the occupation seems free from hazard, exposure in the home to cosmetics, soaps, detergents and plants must be explored.

Previous treatment

Local applications may have been home remedies, proprietary or prescribed medicines but will always have modified the appearance of the eruption, for better or worse.

Differential diagnosis from atopic eczema

Atopic eczema is the commonest differential diagnosis. The history is often of greater help than the appearance. Atopic eczema is suggested by a history of eczema in infancy, eczema of the hands starting before leaving school or the onset of eczema in the popliteal fossae and antecubital fossae, spreading to other areas. Hay fever or asthma may accompany the eruption and there may be a family history of eczema, asthma or hay fever. While these factors make a diagnosis of atopic eczema more probable, this does not exclude superimposed contact dermatitis.

Clinical features

The appearance depends on the acuteness of the eruption, its severity and the site. It rapidly progresses from erythema to papule and vesicle formation, scaling and eventually exudation and oedema. On the palm, vesicles remain intact and may become large, tense blisters sometimes secondarily infected. Dermatitis is chronic when it is scaly, lichenfied, excoriated and fissured.

TYPES OF DERMATITIS

Irritant or traumatic dermatitis

Irritant dermatitis is commoner than allergic contact dermatitis and is responsible for about 70% of cases of industrial dermatitis. Inert dusts, such as coal and stone dust, glass wool and some cements damage the epidermis by abrasion, usually in areas in contact with clothing. Some chemicals cause damage if in contact with the skin in sufficient concentration for long enough. Strong acids and alkalis produce epidermal necrosis within hours, but the effect of detergents is cumulative and may take weeks or months to produce dermatitis.

Allergic contact dermatitis

The incidence is low, accounting for only 14% of all industrial dermatitis. Many substances handled at home or in industry can produce specific immunological hypersensitivity. The capacity of most chemicals for causing sensitization depends upon their concentration, the length of time in contact and the previous susceptibility.

Patch tests Patch tests differentiate irritant from allergic dermatitis. They confirm the diagnosis by application of the suspected allergen to the patient's skin in a concentration which would produce no reaction if the patient were not sensitized. The tests are read at 48 and 96 hours. A typical positive result is shown in Figure 8.1. Patch tests should not be carried out in severe or widespread dermatitis as they may exacerbate the condition and produce misleading results.

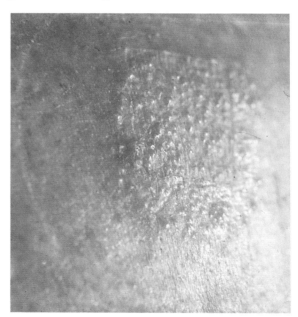

Fig. 8.1 Positive patch test.

It is usual to patch test at a 1% concentration of the suspect substance but this may need to be diluted to 0.1% to be sure that it is a sensitizer and not a primary irritant. If the chemical constituents are known or can be determined, tables from a standard work can be used to check the concentration and diluent for the test.

Substances manufactured to be used on the skin have been tested by the manufacturers so it is reasonable to use them undiluted. Plant leaves can be used but it is important to know which plants are being applied as some are primary irritants unsuitable for patch testing.

When the history points to a cause such as primula or a cosmetic, patch testing can be limited to that substance.

Often the number of substances to be tested is daunting such as with cosmetics or plant sensitivity but it is important to carry out a patch test to them all.

More difficult are cases for which no definite cause can be proved. In these, battery patch tests are useful. Where photo contact dermatitis is suspected, patch tests are duplicated and one set irradiated with long wave, ultra-violet light after 48 hours. The two sets are read after a further 48 hours.

Theoretically, a patch test could sensitize the patient. This occurs infrequently and is no contraindication to diagnostic patch testing in established dermatitis. It is a valid reason for avoiding prospective patch tests in industry.

In suspected clothing dermatitis, patch tests sometimes give unsatisfactory results. The diagnosis is established by asking the patient to observe the results of wearing the suspected garment. If more than one test is positive, it has to be decided if the substance is the primary cause or whether it is secondary.

A common cause of a false positive patch test is the application of an irritant. In some cases many patch tests are positive, with weaker responses around a strongly positive reaction. This is the 'angry back syndrome', an indication to repeat relevant single patch tests.

COMMON CAUSES OF DERMATITIS

Irritant dermatitis

Although strong acids and alkalis obviously irritate or even burn the skin such incidents are fortunately unusual. More common are the insiduous effects of degreasing agents.

Detergents Detergent dermatitis particularly affects young mothers having to wash baby clothes and nappies. Other risk groups are cleaners, home helps and hairdressers.

Hairdressers dermatitis Many who develop irritant dermatitis are atopics, who may have had eczema in childhood and even have been free from trouble for years. They should be warned not to take up work exposing their hands to irritants. Their skin breaks down more easily than normal and the recurrence of their hand eczema often persists when they give up work.

Hairdressing apprentices with traumatic dermatitis, particularly atopics, are best advised to give up the work before they develop chronic hand eczema. Established hairdressers are more likely to become sensitized but may continue to work by using topical corticosteroids and avoiding the offending substance.

Degreasing agents   Trichlorethylene, paraffin, paint thinners and similar compounds are used by engineers and electricians. It should always be possible to avoid coming into contact with the substance. Gloves are not always worn and are not necessarily of the correct type, as solvents penetrate most types of glove, polyvinyl chloride providing the least protection, neoprene and nitriles being the most effective. People removing paint from the hands with thinners or cleaning hands with paraffin have a high risk of developing dermatitis (Fig. 8.2).

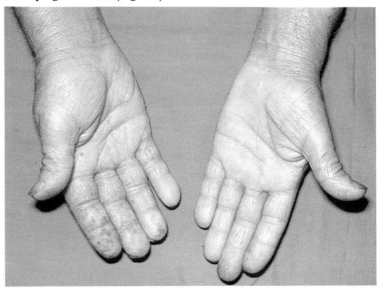

Fig. 8.2   Irritant dermatitis due to degreasing agents such as carbon tetrachloride (courtesy of Dr I B Sneddon).

Soluble cutting oils   The commonest problem caused by soluble cutting oils is primary irritant contact dermatitis. They contain soaps as emulsifiers and are invariably alkaline. Faulty dilution or addition of common soda as a rust inhibitor may increase the alkalinity and cause dermatitis, especially in winter months. Rust inhibitors such as hydroxylamines and nitrites are also potential irritants. Contamination of machine sumps may lead to bacterial overgrowth which gradually decompose the emulsion and added bactericides may be responsible for outbreaks of sensitization dermatitis. Some oils contain anti-oxidants which may sensitize. Dyes and perfumes in the oil may cause problems.

Coolants   Chemical coolants which contain little or no oil are even more alkaline and contain corrosion inhibitors. They are primary irritants and must be diluted accurately. Hardened steels contain nickel, chrome and cobalt. Salts formed during machining may cause sensitization dermatitis.

It is not safe to use gloves as they may be caught in the machinery. The flow of coolant often continues when the machine has been stopped so that hands are wet with the coolant for much of the day. Dermatitis starts as increasing dryness of the skin which progresses to eczema over the finger webs and the backs of the hands, fingers and wrists. This improves when away from work and relapses on return.

A change in working practice and treatment often controls the condition. Affected persons may need to move to another machine or to change the type of coolant or, if possible, to wear gloves. Local corticosteroids have greatly improved the prognosis and this type of dermatitis is helped by the use of conditioning creams at the end of the day.

Allergic dermatitis

Allergic contact dermatitis has a different outlook from that of the irritant state. Continued contact with the sensitizer, however brief, leads to increasingly severe dermatitis and can only be improved by removal from the offending agent.

Nickel
Nickel is the commonest sensitizer in women, the main source being cheap jewellery. Nickel sensitivity in men is most obvious in platers, often affecting the eyelids before involving other exposed areas. Scissors, coins, cutlery, taps and door knobs are all potential sources and, at work, nickel may be leached out in cutting oils. Watches and strap buckles are also a likely source.

Strict avoidance of nickel-containing metals is vital to recovery. This is particularly true of nickel plated clips and fasteners on clothing even if separated from the skin by clothing. A layer of nail varnish or liquid polyurethane plastic is not satisfactory for coating clothing clips as it tends to chip. Nickel plated objects in the home which cannot be replaced easily may usefully be coated in this fashion.

Doubt whether a metal contains nickel may be settled by the dimethylglyoxime spot test. A drop of a 1% alcoholic solution of dimethylglyoxime is placed on the object and a few drops of ammonia added. If nickel is present, the solution turns pink.

Oral ingestion of nickel may play a part in perpetuating hand eczema. Where all else fails a low nickel diet may be worth trying. Canned and acid foods cooked in stainless steel utensils must be avoided, as should food with high nickel content. The role of chelating agents in preventing nickel dermatitis has not been fully evaluated. Improvement has been described on ethylenediamine-tetra-acetic acid (EDTA), and after disulfiram, 200 mg daily for 8 weeks.

Cobalt
Cobalt sensitivity occurs with nickel sensitivity in women and with chromate sensitivity in men, reaction to cobalt alone being unusual.

Chromate
Chromate dermatitis is usually occupational among men, in cement workers, metal workers and offset lithographers. Among women, bleach

containing sodium dichromate and detergents is the sensitizer. In both sexes, the chrome in leather causes shoe dermatitis.

Cement   Dermatitis is common among cement workers. Cement dries and cracks the hands, most frequently in those new to handling it. The skin usually hardens and the condition improves. Prolonged contact with wet cement, particularly when kneeling, can cause alkaline burns. The chromate and cobalt content of cements can cause allergic dermatitis. In over 50% of cases, cement dermatitis is on the hands and arms but it may spread to the trunk as large sheets of weeping eczema or to the limbs as discoid eczema. 80% of building workers with dermatitis have been reported to react to chromate.

The chromium in cement is water-soluble in the alkaline cement and is therefore potentially sensitizing. Trivalent chromium is insoluble in alkali and less likely to sensitize. Adding ferrous sulphate to the cement during mixing converts the chromium to an insoluble form and could help to prevent dermatitis.

Cement dermatitis heals in a significant number of cases despite continued contact, but changing the job may not necessarily improve the prognosis. In many cases, the dermatitis is not very disabling and people can continue working, controlling the skin with topical corticosteroids and short periods off work.

Because of the difficulties of avoiding chrome, attempts have been made to produce a chemical barrier cream. A combination of sodium pyrosulphate and tartaric acid has been effective.

Cosmetics   If the history of the results of the patch testing point towards cosmetic dermatitis, the patient should stop using all cosmetics. They should take all their cosmetics to the clinic, whether or not they have been using them for years, because it is possible to develop sensitization at any time. The number of substances is sometimes daunting but it is important to carry out patch tests to them all. If sensitivity is proved, the offending cosmetic should be discarded. It may be necessary to discard all cosmetics from the same manufacturer as they often contain a common perfume. In some cases it may be necessary to advise the use of hypo-allergenic cosmetics.

Epoxy resins   Epoxy resins have probably caused more industrial dermatitis than any other new chemical. They are used in adhesives, surface coatings and paints, and in the electrical and construction industries. Hardened epoxy resin is non-allergenic but it can remain unhardened for many months if left to harden at room temperature. The hands may be affected if unprotected but more characteristically, when gloves have been worn, it first affects the eyelids, then spreads over exposed areas of the face and neck. The genitalia may also be affected.

Once resin sensitivity is established it persists and it is therefore necessary to remove the worker from any exposure. The main part of management is therefore prevention.

Acrylates   Methyl methacrylate has been used for many years in dentures and can cause dermatitis among dentists and dental technicians. The incidence has greatly diminished, probably due to greater care in handling. Light-sensitive acrylates have also caused dermatitis in printers.

Rubber   Rubber itself is harmless but in manufacturing processes chemicals are added.

In industry and in the home, PVC gloves can be substituted for rubber in most jobs. Surgeons and laboratory technicians can substitute Puritee gloves.*

Shoe dermatitis   The dermatitis is either confined to the weight-bearing area of the sole which may be the only contact with the sensitizer, or it may produce the pattern of the upper part of the shoe on the dorsum of the foot.

In children, glazed, slightly scaly and sometimes fissured juvenile plantar dermatosis appears on the plantar aspect of the toes and the distal sole. This is difficult to distinguish from shoe dermatitis but in children under the age of puberty patch tests are nearly always negative. This is thought to be due to the occlusive effect of synthetic fabrics in socks and shoes.

Insist on seeing all the patient's shoes and slippers. Thin slices of the material from the appropriate parts should be applied as patch tests. Potassium dichromate, the rubber chemicals and shoe and stocking dyes should also be applied. When the offending agent is identified, shoe companies may advise on shoes without sensitizer. Rarely, patients may need hand-made shoes. In such cases, the patient should have patch tests to the ingredients before they are made.

Formaldehyde   Urea formaldehyde resins are used to produce crease resistance in clothes. For the very sensitive, clothing can be tested for formaldehyde. The clothes containing it can be discarded. The patient should avoid drip and crease resistant clothes and wash new clothes before wearing them.

Occupational formaldehyde sensitivity occurs in staff working in pathology and renal units, and in embalmers. Hairdressers may be in contact with formaldehyde in shampoos, printers when it is used as a preservative in offset printing, and urea formaldehyde resin or formaldehyde itself is found in some types of paper.

Phosphorus pentasulphide   This is contained in strike-anywhere matches and has caused dermatitis for over 50 years. The subjects, usually men, have attacks of facial dermatitis, especially on the eyelids or the muzzle area and occasionally on the hands. If they carry the box in a trouser pocket the patch of dermatitis on one thigh confirms the diagnosis. Phosphorus pentasulphide sometimes seems to be a mild irritant but the patch test can be carried out with the crushed head of the match.

*Manufactured by Searle and Medical Products, PO Box 88, Lane End Road, High Wycombe, Bucks, England, or Elastyren gloves (manufactured by Danpren A/S 272, Vigeislevvej, DK 2500, Valvy, Denmark).

Paraphenylinediamine   This is widely used as a hair dye. Those sensitive to it may develop cross-reaction to antihistamines and azo dyes. Industrial exposure occurs in hairdressers, furriers, leather processors, printers and lithographers.

Instruction for patch tests to the dye may be included on the container label. Patch testing is often overlooked in those having their hair dyed regularly.

Plants   Compositae, primulae and plants of the Liliaceae family are the commonest sensitizers. Chrysanthemums are the most troublesome. The dermatitis affects the exposed areas of the skin over the face, neck, forearms and hands, suggesting an airborne allergen, easily mistaken for light sensitivity.

Primula lesions consist of streaky papules and vesicles on the fingers (Fig. 8.3), forearms and sometimes the face. They last for 1–2 days then dry up and peel off only to appear elsewhere in proximal areas. Poison Ivy dermatitis in the USA looks like a giant version of primula dermatitis with bullae rather than vesicles. Sufferers can be so severely affected that they may need systemic steroids.

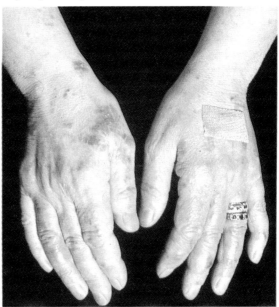

Fig. 8.3   Contact sensitization dermatitis due to Primula obconica (courtesy of Dr I. B. Sneddon).

Tulips and garlic cause chronic dermatitis of the finger tips.

In many cases the diagnosis is obvious. Patients need to bring a leaf of all the plants to which they are exposed for patch testing, each in a separate labelled envelope. Some may be primary irritants and unsuitable for patch testing. The buttercup family is an example.

Coolant oils   Continued contact with coolant oil, however brief, can lead to an increasingly severe dermatitis that will improve only on removal from the offending agent.

It is necessary to establish which chemical in the coolant is the cause and to persuade the employer to change the coolant for one which does not contain it. Even then, dermatitis may still not settle completely and may relapse in a non-specific way on any contact with coolants.

Hairdressers   Allergic dermatitis is less common in hairdressers than irritant dermatitis and may be caused by nickel, rubber,formaldehyde, paraphenylinediamine (PPD) and other hair dyes.

Phototoxic and photoallergic contact dermatitis

Phototoxic dermatitis can affect anyone without previous exposure. The reaction in the skin is mediated by long-wave ultraviolet light (UVA). The commonest is phytophoto dermatitis from exposure to furocoumarine in plants, such as the Umbelliferae (e.g. cow parsley and giant hog weed). In skin which has been in contact with the plant, particularly on a damp, sunny day, streaks of acute dermatitis appear which may blister quite severely. They subside but the streaks persist as hyper-pigmentation for some weeks. Coal tar derivatives may also cause a phototoxic eruption

Photoallergic contact dermatitis does not occur on first exposure, but after several days. Antibacterial halogenated phenols (especially tetrachlorosalicylanilide) in soaps and cosmetics have caused light-sensitive dermatitis. Sporadic cases of light sensitivity are ascribed to currently available substances such as hexachlorophene and phenothiazines.

Photoallergic dermatitis produces confluent erythema over the light exposed areas, mainly of the face, neck, V area, forearms, backs of the hands and, in women, the lower legs. It usually resolves rapidly when the sensitizing agent is withdrawn and the patient keeps out of direct sunshine but occasional cases remain light sensitive for months or even years. They may need a light barrier cream in the summer.

INDUSTRIAL DERMATITIS

Many of the substances which may be involved have been discussed above in the irritant and allergic dermatitis sections. Some appear in both. The following relates to considerations concerning industrial dermatitis.

Prognosis in industrial dermatitis

The prognosis in industrial dermatitis is greatly improved if it is recognised early, the subject removed from the cause and the outbreak treated. Repeated attacks often lead to chronic and intractable dermatitis.

Traumatic dermatitis is more likely to occur in the over-40s and to become chronic. Age also affects the possibilities of re-training. It has generally a better prognosis than sensitivity dermatitis but this depends on the type of sensitivity.

Those sensitive to primulae or epoxy resins can easily avoid them and should have no further skin trouble. Rubber should be easy to avoid though some find it very hard to do so. Chromate and nickel are almost impossible to avoid so that the prognosis is bad for nickel and chromium dermatitis of the hands. In atopic subjects with hand eczema due to exposure to irritants, the prognosis is that of the underlying eczema.

The outlook is best if the worker can remain in the same job. This is usually possible in traumatic dermatitis when it is controlled and protective measures prevent further trauma. In specific sensitivities, such as to epoxy resins, the worker has to move away from the substance to another part of the factory with no risk of contamination. Coolant oils can be changed. The worst option is for him to stop his work and be labelled as a dermatitis case, as employers will be reluctant to take him on in any other job in case they are blamed for a recurrence.

Other occupational dermatoses

Contact urticaria Contact urticaria, i.e. the weal and flare response can occur without previous sensitization, to a number of chemical irritants, such as benzoic acid, cinnamic acid and cinnamic aldehyde.

Cinammon is found mainly in toothpastes and chewing gum and benzoic acid in skin creams as a preservative. Rubefacients such as nicotinic acid for muscle and joint strains may produce urticaria, as may persulphates in hairdressers.

Allergic contact urticaria is commoner in atopic subjects after stroking cats or dogs, or handling foods. The occupational form is most common in food handlers. Fish, shellfish, onions, garlic, cheese, potatoes and apples are the main food causes. An open prick patch test confirms the diagnosis. Small squares of the foods are placed on the flexor aspect of the forearm and the skin pricked through the food with a needle. After 20 minutes the skin is inspected for a reaction.

Occupational vitiligo In vitiligo, patches of skin form white, ringed or irregular serpiginous areas, usually symmetrical, but they retain their normal texture. This is due to a reduction in the number or complete absence of normal melanocytes. It affects about 1% of the total population and is usually idiopathic.

Some chemicals obliterate melanocytes and produce depigmentation indistinguishable from idiopathic vitiligo. The onset of vitiligo in several workers in a chemical factory should suggest an occupational origin. Chemicals implicated are found in neoprene adhesive, oil anti-oxidants and germicides in detergents.

Occupational vitiligo usually remains static, or may even worsen after removal from contact with the offending chemical. Any later repigmentation is rarely complete.

Oil acne

With poor hygiene the pilo-sebaceous follicle is irritated by oil. Neat cutting oils and greases are the usual cause but any oil, including vegetable oil, can produce the lesions. It may occur wherever oily clothes rub. Better hygiene is essential. Oil-proof sleevelets and aprons protect against it. The lesions subside spontaneously, although slowly.

Chloracne

Chlorinated hydrocarbons in industrial synthetic wax may produce an acne-like eruption over the malar areas of the face and temples, though it can spread wider. Recently even more troublesome acne has affected people exposed to chlorodibenzodioxine, usually after accidental spillage. The amounts needed to cause it are so small that even the families of chemical workers have been affected by the amounts taken home on the clothes.

No treatment seems effective but removal from the chemical is followed by very slow improvement over several years, sometimes leaving pitted scarring.

Occupational cancer

Exposure to tar, pitch and bitumen is probably the commonest occupational cause of skin cancer. Exposed skin becomes hyper-pigmented with scattered keratoses, developing years later into squamous carcinomata. Ultraviolet light produces the carcinogenic effect so that workers could be protected by a light barrier cream.

Carcinoma is only likely to be found in older men exposed in the past to unrefined oils.

Chronic absorption of arsenic leads to multiple squamous cell carcinomata, skin pigmentation and keratoses on palms and soles. Occupational exposure to arsenic is rare but may occur in the manufacture of sheep dips and insecticides.

Pigmentation

Increased melanin pigmentation is common in tar and pitch workers because of their increased sensitivity to light. Mists of cutting oils may induce reticulate pigmentation with telangiectasia and atrophy of the exposed skin. Some silversmiths still get argyria, a slate grey colouration of the skin and sclera. It is harmless.

Chrome ulcers

Alkaline hexavalent chromate solutions produce indolent ulcers at the sites of trauma, and on the nasal septum, in tanners, electroplaters and workers in the chrome industry. Better hygiene has made them rare. An ointment of 10% edathamil calcium, a chelating agent, has been used, but the ulcers heal spontaneously in time.

MANAGEMENT OF DERMATITIS—GENERAL MEASURES

Management of some specific conditions has been discussed under the name of the appropriate substance. The following are general considerations applicable to the home and industry.

The aim is to prevent contact of any potential irritant or sensitizer but in practice this is not always possible; the risk must be minimised by whatever means necessary. In the home it is largely a matter of gloves and the housewife should be encouraged to wear lined PVC rather than rubber gloves.

In industry, prevention is more complex. The means used may be the subject of legislation; often prevention can never be complete and may be the subject of litigation.

Selection of personnel

Atopic eczema sufferers and those with a history of atopic eczema are more prone to traumatic dermatitis if exposed to irritants. People with a history of dermatitis of the hands should not be placed in jobs exposed to irritants. The same applies to ichthyosis, in which the skin is more easily degreased. Prospective patch testing is useless and carries a risk of sensitization.

Barrier creams

Barrier creams do nothing to prevent allergic dermatitis. Proponents claim that they make cleansing easier but any advantage is minimal. The use of barrier creams under ordinary gloves should be discouraged. Oil repellant barrier creams often contain soap and under occlusion can produce dermatitis. Applied as a patch test they may give a false positive result from their irritant reaction.

Conditioning creams

The application of an emollient after cleaning the hands is to be encouraged and probably does more to prevent traumatic dermatitis than applying a barrier cream beforehand.

Topical corticosteroids

In most contact dermatitis, local corticosteroids effectively suppress the eruption. As the hands are the most commonly affected area and penetration of the thickened hand skin by corticosteroids is slow, full strength corticosteroid applications should be used. Dermatitis of the face and eyelids responds to hydrocortisone ointments twice daily. Widespread involvement of the trunk and limbs, either from contact with fabrics or as a sensitization spread, should be treated with a low potency corticosteroid twice daily. Severely affected patients should rest in bed until it subsides.

A blistering dermatitis on the hands is often secondarily infected. Initially treatment is with wet dressings of 0.5% Silver Nitrate Lotion or Eusol to the hands two or three times daily, and an appropriate antibiotic. Erythromycin 250 mg four times a day for a week is usually adequate. Large bullae on the hands should be snipped open. When the blisters subside and the hands begin to dry, a steroid ointment containing an antibiotic such as aureomycin can be applied twice daily. Patch tests should be avoided in acute dermatitis as they may produce a focal flare.

The treatment of chronic dermatitis also mainly relies on corticosteroid ointments or creams in sufficient concentration, twice daily, to bring it under control. Soap should be avoided and emulsifying ointment used as a substitute. Where topical steroids on their own fail to control chronic dermatitis, polythene occlusion at night is useful, using disposable polythene gloves for hands and thin plastic film (Clingfilm, Saranwrap®) held in place with adhesive tape for the limbs. Occlusion should not be continued for more than 10–14 days because of the risk of infection and skin atrophy.

Other measures

Chronic cases tend to behave like endogenous eczema and if topical corticosteroids are unsuccessful, a crude coal tar preparation is sometimes useful. It should be applied at night under tube-gauze or cotton gloves and cleaned off in the morning with liquid paraffin. A topical corticosteroid cream is used during the day. Very resistant cases may respond to coal tar paste bandages left on for weekly periods.

Where these measures fail and the patient is incapacitated by dermatitis, superficial X-ray therapy to the affected areas can control it, giving 100 R at 40 kv on three occasions at two-week intervals. Improvement may be expected about a month after the last dose.

Systemic treatment

Antihistamines have no direct effect on the course of dermatitis but control the pruritus. If the patient is still at work, terfenadine 60 mg twice daily relieves itching without causing undue drowsiness. Hydroxyzine in divided doses of 25–75 mg daily also controls itching but may make the subject dangerously drowsy. Systemic steroids are hardly ever indicated though rhus dermatitis (Poison Ivy) in America can produce a severe and prolonged bullous eruption and may merit them. Occasional cases of contact dermatitis produce severe and generalised erythroderma which may progress to exfoliative dermatitis, for which systemic steroids should be used, unless there are serious contra-indications. Prednisone 30 mg daily should be given until the skin has settled. It can then be slowly reduced by 5 mg every 3 days.

FURTHER READING

Cronin E 1980 Contact dermatitis. Churchill Livingstone, Edinburgh
Fisher A A 1973 Contact dermatitis, 2nd ed. Lea and Febiger, Philadelphia
Griffiths W A D 1985 Essentials of industrial dermatology, Blackwell Scientific
    Publications, London

P. A. Dufton

9. Psoriasis

Clinical features 1.5–2% of the population have psoriasis. The cause is unknown although there appears to be a genetic link and the whole process of epidermal cell turnover is accelerated. Many never present to the doctor, probably unaware that they have psoriasis, mistakenly thinking that they have dandruff or abnormal nails. A few have such severe psoriasis that they are virtually never clear. Some are so severely affected that it is the cause of their death. In the middle are many people with chronic psoriasis which responds extremely well to traditional treatments (with a variety of drawbacks).

Management Many doctors tell their patients they have psoriasis because of stress and worry. They should not be given psychotropic drugs for their psoriasis, as they make no difference to the disease. Many are very upset, anxious and stressful, and relaxation therapy may help some of them. There is an element of faith in the treatment. The patient should realise that the doctor is confident in the knowledge that the treatment will make him or her better. It is no good saying 'look, you have psoriasis, you have to live with it.' Certainly he has to live with it but with the help of treatment.

Psoriatics also ask about sunbeds. Some find they are slightly improved and they certainly tan, which makes them feel better, but it is not a specific treatment for psoriasis. Some are greatly improved if they go on holiday. This may be due to a combination of the helpful effects of ultra-violet light and the fact that they are resting and relaxing.

CHRONIC PLAQUE-TYPE PSORIASIS

Clinical features The psoriatic lesion is characterized by silvery scales on well-demarcated reddened plaque-like areas of the skin, particularly on the back of the elbows and the front of the knees. It may involve almost the whole of the body, including the scalp. Psoriasis is aggravated by such events as injury to the skin, acute infection, anxiety and certain drugs such as lithium and antimalarials.

Management   For chronic plaque-type psoriasis (Fig. 9.1) the best treatment with the longest remission time is dithranol, second best is coal tar. Even without treatment, patches of psoriasis come and go. When they begin to clear, they often do so from the centre. Treatment of chronic psoriasis is highly likely to be successful.

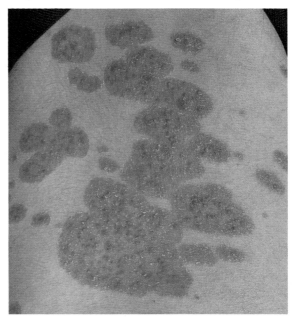

Fig. 9.1 Chronic plaque-type psoriasis.

Dithranol, commonly in Lassar's paste, is applied to each plaque (Fig. 9.2). Application takes about one hour in skilled dermatological nursing hands if the eruption is very extensive, a very big drawback. The fact that it has to be carefully applied to the lesions to prevent burning of normal skin is another. Lassar's paste will not wash off and this is also a great drawback. In the ward the paste is hardened further by applying talcum powder so that it does not spread when it is warm. Tube gauze dressings will also minimise spreading. The aim is to produce staining on the skin around the lesion (Fig. 9.3). Only normal skin stains; once the patient is covered in stains his psoriasis has gone. In the Ingram technique each application of dithranol in Lassar's paste is preceded by a tar bath and exposure to ultra-violet light (UVB).

Unfortunately, dithranol stains clothing, bedding, cast iron bedsteads and the floor beneath the beds. The whole ward is permanently stained with dithranol. Stains will peel off patients and disappear in about 7−10 days after stopping treatment.

Dithranol is slightly caustic and if the skin is burnt too much by an inappropriately high concentration, the psoriasis will worsen. It is normal to start at 0.1% to go up to 0.25%, and then 0.5%.

The modern proprietary dithranol cream preparations are much more convenient for outpatients. They are extremely good, well tolerated, have an increasing range of concentrations and wash off easily. They still stain

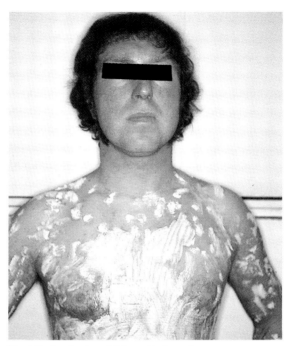

Fig. 9.2 Application of dithranol in Lassar's paste.

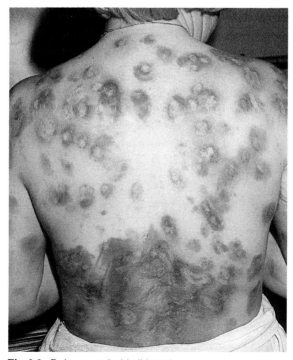

Fig. 9.3 Patient treated with dithranol.

clothing however and the staining is worse in the presence of alkali. All detergents are alkaline so if patients soak the clothes first for 24 hours in cold water the staining is reduced but not abolished.

The patient must be told that unless there is staining, the treatment is not working. If there is no staining the preparation is not strong enough or is not being used. The patient cannot tell you that he is using dithranol when he is not. The staining may be removed more quickly by applying 2% salicylic acid in white soft paraffin or oily cream. Dithranol staining can be a big disadvantage, particularly on the backs of the hands or the face; some are surprised when they come in for the first time covered with psoriasis and go out covered with brown stains. They do not necessarily think it a great advance. Patients with any skin disease are conscious of their appearance and are not keen on treatment which makes it look worse.

The modern trend for dithranol is to use short contact therapy. The strength is increased to 1% or 5% in white soft paraffin but it is used for a much shorter time, say for half an hour. The ointment is applied, left for 30 minutes, the excess wiped off with paper towels, the area washed with an alkaline soap followed by a shower. All active skin preparations penetrate inflamed skin much more quickly than normal skin. There is ample opportunity for the dithranol to penetrate the psoriatic plaque in 30 minutes and produce its therapeutic effect.

Coal tar ointment, in concentrations up to 10%, is often used as part of the Goeckerman technique. It is applied to the plaques for 24 hours, after which the excess is wiped off and the patient exposed to ultra-violet light (UVB). The remaining traces are removed by bathing.

Nail psoriasis is difficult. There is no effective treatment (see Ch. 20).

FACE AND FLEXURES

Some textbooks state that psoriasis does not occur on the face; this is wrong. It is less common on the face than on other areas. Perhaps ultra-violet light has some beneficial effect.

Dithranol is generally not suitable for treating the face and flexures. The staining produced on the face is cosmetically unacceptable and, if rubbed into the eyes, a severe irritant conjunctivitis is produced.

The flexures must also be treated with caution (Fig. 9.4). The combination of a thinner epidermis, increased temperature and humidity allow dithranol to penetrate more quickly (as of course would steroid preparations) and, therefore, burning with dithranol is much more likely. If used, dithranol should be applied for a shorter period, starting with 2 hours, then going up to 4 hours, followed by a bath to wash it off.

In sites such as these where tar or dithranol are not tolerated so well, topical steroids may be useful; also in inflamed psoriasis or where there are mixed features of eczema. Treatment should not be prolonged and once an effect has been achieved it should be tailed-off gradually.

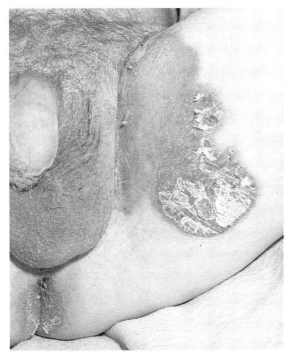

Fig. 9.4 Flexural psoriasis.

PSORIASIS OF THE SCALP

Clinical features It is different simply because scalp hair gets in the way of therapy. The scale is held down by the hair.

Management The best way to apply treatment to the scalp should be explained because patients do not find it obvious. A parting should be made at one side, the ointment applied then another parallel parting about half-an-inch away and so on across the scalp. The ointment is left on overnight if possible or at least for 2 hours and then shampooed out.

To get the pharmacological preparation into the skin, the crust must be removed, and no simple, cosmetically acceptable preparation works. Traditional therapies with salicyclic acid and coal tar have to be used for 1–2 weeks at the beginning of treatment. Several preparations remove scales very well. Routinely 2% salicyclic acid with 10% coal tar solution in emulsifying ointment is applied overnight and washed out in the morning. In more severe scaling, more vigorous preparations may be used, such as 10% oil of cade in arachis oil or pyrogallol compound ointment. It need only be used for 2 weeks before changing to a more cosmetically acceptable effective preparation. After starting the salicylic acid and coal tar preparation patients are often so much better 2 weeks later that they do not want to change. One proprietary dithranol cream can be applied to the scalp overnight and washed out the following day. If anything stronger is needed, one has to change to a different preparation. Shampoos are of very little use because they are in contact with the skin for only a rather short time. However, coal tar shampoos are very suitable for psoriasis. Once the scalp is in a reasonable condition a steroid application is provided. There is no point in using topical steroid lotions prior to this when there is a great amount of scaling because the scalp application will simply sit on the surface.

GUTTATE PSORIASIS

Clinical features   Some forms of psoriasis pose special problems. Guttate psoriasis (Fig. 9.5) is acute and often occurs in children after a streptococcal sore throat. It is very easily irritated. As a result of the Koebner phenomenon, surgical or other trauma, or over-exposure to ultra-violet light may exacerbate the condition.

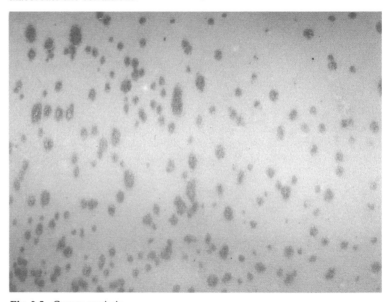

Fig. 9.5 Guttate psoriasis.

Management   In the eruptive phase which lasts for up to 6 weeks, active treatment may make the condition worse and a soothing cream, for example oily cream or a moisturizer, is all that is needed. The condition may continue to erupt and become more chronic, the patches joining together. Active treatment should be considered at about 6–8 weeks, beginning with coal tar, perhaps with tar baths and ultra-violet light if the patient can attend the hospital, or low-concentration dithranol.

CHRONIC PUSTULAR PSORIASIS OF HANDS AND SOLES

Clinical features   Another difficult thereapeutic area is chronic pustular psoriasis of the palms and soles, with its pustules and small brown spots (Fig. 9.6).

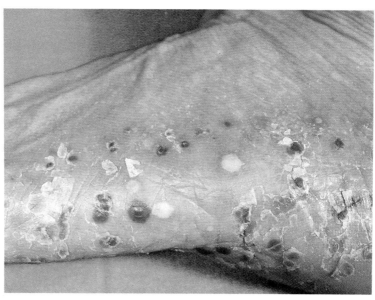

Fig. 9.6 Pustular psoriasis (foot).

These become more typical patches of psoriasis, often with painful fissures.

Management Coal tar overnight (or dithranol) and soft paraffin or a moisturizer during the daytime provide comfort. Occasionally, a topical steroid cream to hands and feet helps when the other treatment has not worked. For a severe case localized photochemotherapy is useful.

GENERALIZED PUSTULAR PSORIASIS AND ERYTHRODERMIC PSORIASIS

Clinical features *Generalized pustular psoriasis* is totally unlike any other form of psoriasis. It occurs occasionally as a result of the withdrawal of systemic steroids or the sudden cessation of treatment with large quantities of topical steroids. This may result in sheets of pustular psoriasis which peel leaving extremely raw, painful psoriasis.

Chronic psoriasis may suddenly become exfoliative and involve almost all of the body surface. Generalized pustular psoriasis may revert to an erythrodermic form.

Management Generalized pustular psoriasis and generalized erythrodermic psoriasis, owing to the severe thermoregulatory and metabolic consequences of total skin inflammation, need vigorous treatment in hospital. Cardiac failure may be precipitated in the elderly. Patients require bed rest with attention to fluid and electrolyte balance as necessary. Bland emollients should be applied to the skin. Methotrexate, which can be given orally, intramuscularly or intravenously, or photochemotherapy is required.

DNA antagonists such as methotrexate reduce epidermopoiesis to normal.

Methotrexate is toxic to bone marrow, gonads and intestinal mucosa and may result in leukopenia and severe systemic infections which may be fatal. It is also hepatotoxic and may give rise to nausea. Thus, patients need regular haematological and biochemical investigations and should have a liver biopsy after each cumulative dose to exclude hepatic damage, leading eventually to cirrhosis. Methotrexate may give rise to female sterility or foetal abnormality and should not be used until after the reproductive years, other than in exceptionally severe cases.

For the dosage of methotrexate see Formulary.

PHOTOCHEMOTHERAPY (PUVA)

High intensity UVA at 360 nm is capable of penetrating to the basal cell layer. Patients are given 8-methoxypsoralens systemically and 2 hours later exposed to a controlled dose of UVA (Figs. 9.7 and 9.8). The drug reacts in the skin with UVA to produce a thymidine antagonist. Increasing amounts of ultra-violet light are administered each week. It is very easy to burn the patient and so treatment has to be strictly monitored. There is a slight worry about stimulating malignancy since ultra-violet light produces solar keratoses, squamous carcinomata and

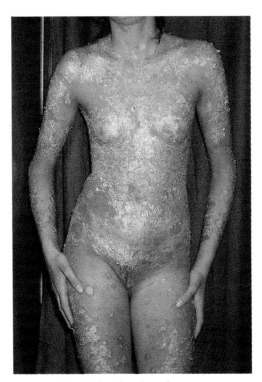

Fig. 9.7 Patient before photochemotherapy.

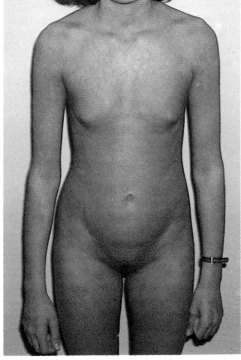

Fig. 9.8 Patient after photochemotherapy.

rodent ulcers, after prolonged therapy. It is therefore not without hazard and should be avoided in childhood and pregnancy.

RETINOIDS

The retinoids etretinate and 13-cis retinoic acid are used in severe extensive psoriasis. Side-effects include loss of some hair, severe soreness of the lips, eyes, nose and cracking of the skin, and skin fragility generally. This may not be ideal but seems safer than drugs such as methotrexate and may well be the treatment of the future. However, it is important to remember that these drugs are teratogenic and should not be prescribed unless precautions are taken to prevent pregnancy (see Ch. 22).

ARTHROPATHY

This occurs in psoriasis and is normally treated in the same way as any other arthritis (Fig. 9.9). The commonest form is identical to rheumatoid arthritis with less tendency to be symmetrical. Rheumatoid factor is negative. The terminal interphalangeal joint is commonly involved and sacroiliitis is often present. Ankylosing spondylitis is rare and arthritis mutilans least common. Finger joints alone may be affected with or without skin involvement in these areas.

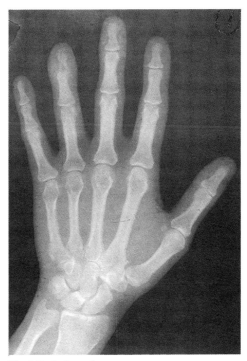

Fig. 9.9 Arthropathy.

S. Evans

10. Erythema Multiforme, Toxic Erythemata, Drug Reactions

ERYTHEMA MULTIFORME

Clinical features   Erythema multiforme is an acute polymorphic eruption. Starting as a maculopapular rash, it progresses to a ringed erythema showing a 'target' appearance as it spreads centrifugally (Fig. 10.1). The edge is pink but the centre may become purplish or purpuric, vesicles or frank bullae appearing in it. It is termed Stevens-Johnson syndrome when the bullous reaction involves mucous membranes of the mouth, eyes and genitalia.

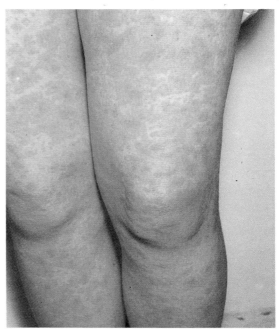

Fig. 10.1   Erythema multiforme. The typical 'target' or 'iris' lesions.

The cause is unknown but appears to be a reaction to circulating immune complexes produced by viruses, bacteria and drugs. Erythema multiforme may complicate pregnancy and rare systemic diseases such as lupus erythematosus, leukaemia and sarcoidosis. The feet, hands, forearms and knees and less commonly the face and neck are affected.

Lesions appear in crops over a few days and last 10 days before fading and leaving pigmentation. There may be mild pyrexia and pruritus.

Stevens-Johnson syndrome is a severe illness, with pyrexia, lymphadenopathy and polyarthritis. The oral ulceration denudes the buccal mucosa. There is haemorrhagic crusting on the lips, catarrhal or purulent conjunctivitis, corneal ulceration and, rarely, panophthalmitis. Genital lesions may result in retention of urine. There may be a more widespread erythema, as well as the typical 'iris' or 'target' lesions.

The commonest provocative factor is herpes simplex infection but other viruses and mycoplasma infections have been implicated. The bacterial organism most often incriminated is the streptococcus.

Drugs, especially barbiturates, sulphonamides, hydantoins and penicillins, may produce erythema multiforme.

Management   In straightforward erythema multiforme, a local antipruritic such as hydrocortisone cream 0.5% with calamine and an oral antihistamine may be all that is needed. Bullous lesions should be 'popped' with a sterile needle and dressed. A local antibiotic cream such as 3% chlortetracycline is suitable for ulcerated lesions, and a systemic antibiotic if they are widespread.

The role of systemic corticosteroids is controversial and may only be indicated for the Stevens-Johnson Syndrome. Prednisolone, 30–60 mg daily may be needed for severe cases tailing off over 10–14 days. Mouth washes incorporating triamcinolone may be all that is necessary, with steroid antibiotic eye drops for any ocular involvement. Lignocaine oral gel is also a useful medication (see Formulary).

When herpes simplex precipitates recurrent attacks of erythema multiforme, topical idoxuridine or acyclovir may abort the attack and prevent the onset of erythema multiforme.

TOXIC ERYTHEMA

Clinical features   Toxic erythema is an exanthematous eruption of rapid onset. Initially confined to the trunk, it tends to spare the face. It presents as a diffuse macular erythema which may become morbilliform or, occasionally, scarlatiniform.

Toxic erythema may be due to a drug reaction or a virus exanthem such as measles, rubella and others.

Erythema infectiosum (fifth disease), and roseola infantum (exanthema subitum) are virus-induced toxic erythemata. The former starts as a ringed erythema on the cheeks (Fig. 10.2), followed by a maculopapular rash on the trunk and limbs. The latter affects children under 2 years of age. After a few days of fever, a maculopapular rash appears on the neck and trunk spreading to the face and limbs. There may be lymphadenopathy.

Drugs which produce toxic erythema include barbiturates, antibiotics, phenylbutazone, thiazides and phenothiazines.

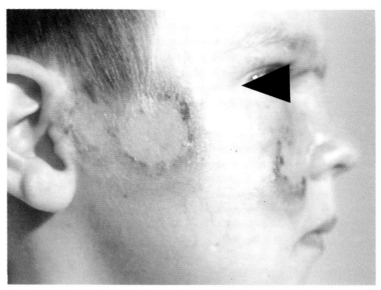

Fig. 10.2 Toxic erythema. The characteristic facial involvement in erythema infectiosum.

Management   Treatment is symptomatic, directed to fluid balance and antipyretics. If a drug cause is suspected it must of course be stopped. Topical calamine lotion or creams and antihistamines may be indicated.

DRUG REACTIONS

Clinically recognisable adverse reactions to drugs are seen more often in the skin than in any other organ or system.

Nearly all drugs may, once in a while, produce an exanthematous type of rash, some often and others rarely. Certain drugs are more likely to cause a particular type of eruption. For example, if a patient taking both demeclocycline and phenothiazine develops photosensitivity the reaction is probably due to the former, although both drugs can cause that particular eruption. If the patient shows hyperpigmentation, the opposite is the case.

Overdosage

Symptoms of overdosage are generally an exaggeration of the normal pharmacological effects, e.g. haemorrhage from anticoagulants—often manifested in the skin. However, the pathogenesis of the bullae in barbiturate intoxication is unclear. Hepatic or renal insufficiency may lead to apparent overdosage especially in the elderly.

Drug interaction may cause serious effects, such as bleeding in a patient on warfarin and aspirin.

Cumulation

One example of this is argyria from the use of silver-containing nasal drops. More typical, perhaps, is the thinning, coarsening and loss of hair with cheilitis and conjunctivitis, from the retinoids. Others include reversible alopecia from cytostatic agents, and excessive sweating from tricyclic antidepressants.

Idiosyncracy and intolerance

Inherited enzyme deficiencies can be a problem, as in patients with glucose-6-phosphate dehydrogenase deficiency who develop haemolytic anaemia on primaquine.

Ecological imbalance

The classical example is candidosis after administration of systemic steroids, broad spectrum antibiotics and cytotoxic drugs.

Exacerbation of existing latent or overt disease

Porphyria can be precipitated by drugs, such as barbiturates, griseofulvin and oral contraceptives. Dermatitis herpetiformis may be exacerbated by iodides and lupus erythematosus may be induced by hydralazine; steroids may worsen pyogenic infections.

Hypersensitivity reactions

Drugs act as complete or incomplete antigens. Impurities in them may also act antigenically. Ampicillin eruptions some years ago were shown to be due to a contaminant, as are probably the rare instances of allergic sensitivity to steroids.

Sensitivity to drugs increases with age and reactions are more frequent in females than males, possibly due to a higher consumption.

Hypersensitivity reactions can be classified into four types:

Type I—Anaphylactic   In a Type I reaction, histamine, heparin and kinins are released from IgE-sensitized mast cells and basophils. Anaphylaxis and urticaria are the result. Massive release of histamine leads to bronchiolar constriction, localized oedema, often in laryngeal and glottal regions, and vasodilation with hypotension and shock.

Type II—Cytotoxic   In this reaction the antigen attaches to cell surfaces, the antigen-antibody IgG or IgM complexes take up complement and the cell is destroyed.

Acute haemolytic anaemia and allergic thrombocytopenic reactions are due to this mechanism.

Type III   Deposition of soluble antigen-antibody IgG or IgM complexes, with the uptake of complement in vessel walls or in basement membranes causes local inflammation.

This is the serum sickness or Arthus reaction. In serum sickness, it takes from 5–14 days to build up antibodies. The patient then develops fever, exanthemata, urticaria, lymphadenopathy and arthralgia, which may last several days or weeks. Vascular lesions may last longer with chronic arterial inflammation, similar to polyarteritis nodosa, particularly in patients continuing to take a sulphonamide. Urticaria is usually an isolated sign of drug hypersensitivity but may be part of serum sickness.

Type IV—Delayed cellular   There are no circulating antibodies in this reaction, but they may be found in lymphocytes. The reaction is delayed for 24–48 hours, the classic example being contact dermatitis. Most exanthemata are delayed cellular reactions.

Autoimmune reactions

Lupus erythematosus and thrombocytopenic purpura fall into this category. The drug may alter auto-antigens in some way, but it is not known if auto-antibodies are the result or the cause of tissue damage.

The above mechanisms do not explain all patterns of drug reactions. The pathogenesis of erythema multiforme, toxic epidermal necrolysis or a fixed drug eruption remains obscure.

Patterns of drug reactions

Acne   Acneiform eruptions are due to a variety of drugs, the commonest being steroids, bromides, iodides and anticonvulsants.

Alopecia   This commonly follows cytotoxic drugs but hormones and antithyroid drugs may be incriminated.

Hyperpigmentation   This is blue-grey, from antimalarials and phenothiazines or brownish from anticonvulsants, cytotoxics, arsenic and metals.

Exanthematous eruptions   These are often seen with penicillins (Fig. 10.3) but they can be caused by other drugs. A first attack starts with fever on about the 9th day of administration. Subsequent attacks start on the 2nd and 3rd day. All penicillins may induce urticaria as an immediate or Type I sensitivity and an exanthematous rash as part of a delayed cellular or Type IV reaction. Not all drug-induced urticarias are allergic. Direct histamine liberators include aspirin, opiates and quinine.

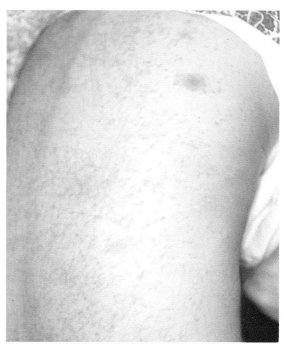

Fig. 10.3 Exanthematous eruption due to cloxacillin.

Eczema Eczema may appear in a patient previously sensitized to a contact allergen. Penicillin and sulphonamides should not be prescribed topically. Cross-sensitivity may occur between the para-amino group and tolbutamide, sulphonamides and chlorpropamide. Eczema may occur, however, from a drug such as methyldopa with no previous relevant cross-sensitivity.

Exfoliative erythroderma This severe skin eruption with fever, malaise, lymphadenopathy and finally hyperpigmentation may follow the pyrazoline drugs, tuberculostatics, gold, streptomycin and others.

Photosensitivity Photosensitivity may be phototoxic which is dose-dependent or photoallergic. Light-exposed areas show anything from a mild erythema to urticaria and acute weeping vesicular eczema.

In some patients a photosensitivity persists after discontinuing the offending drug. Drugs implicated include sulphonamides, tetracyclines, nalidixic acid and chlorothiazides, which can produce a photo-lichenoid eruption (see Ch. 15).

Lupus erythematosus There appears to be a genetic susceptibility in individuals who develop drug-induced lupus. Symptoms usually subside after withdrawal of the drug. 'LE-like syndromes' may follow hydralazine, procainamide, anticonvulsants, methyldopa and thyrostatics (Fig. 10.4).

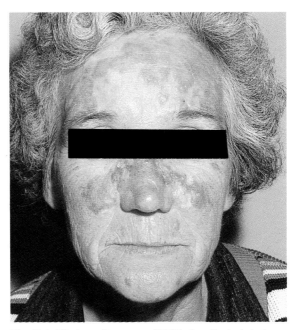

Fig. 10.4   The butterfly pattern of SLE induced by hydralazine.

Vascular reactions   Allergic vasculitis and a polyarteritis nodosa-like syndrome may be drug-induced: sulphonamides, pyrazolones, indomethacin and thiouracils being the most likely culprits.

Erythema nodosum   This involves the larger vessels in the subcutis (Fig. 10.5). Although erythema nodosum due to drugs is rare, oral contraceptives, sulphonamides, salicylates and halogens have been implicated.

Purpura   Frusemide is commonly implicated in drug-induced purpura (Fig. 10.6) but chlorothiazides, sulphonamides, aspirin, quinine, gold and pyrazolones can also cause it.

Porphyria   Porphyria is induced particularly by barbiturates, griseofulvin and the contraceptive pill, but also by any hepatotoxic drug.

Lichenoid drug eruptions   Lichenoid drug eruptions often have a photosensitive component. Thickened and usually pigmented lesions appear on light-exposed areas such as the back of the hand. Antimalarials, gold, dapsone, methyldopa, arsenic, thiazides and chlorpromazine are causes. This reaction is thought to be dose-dependent and is therefore toxic rather than allergic.

A *fixed drug eruption* always occurs at the same site when the drug is ingested. The commonest cause is phenolphthalein (Fig. 10.7); the others include tetracyclines.

Vesico-bullous   This reaction occurs with other eruptions such as urticaria, photosensitivity and severe eczematous rashes, drug-induced porphyrias

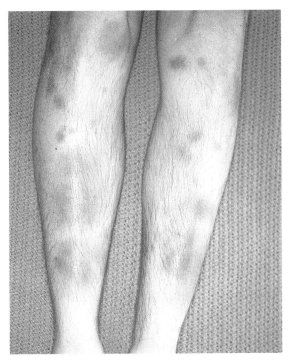

Fig. 10.5   The typical appearances of erythema nodosum.

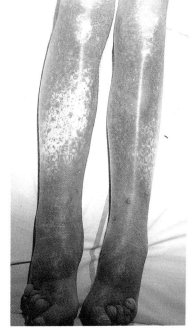

Fig. 10.6   A diffuse purpura due to frusemide.

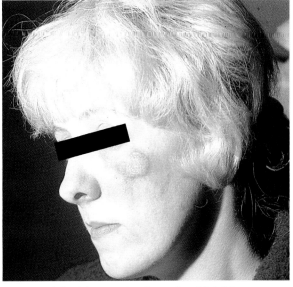

Fig. 10.7   A fixed drug eruption due to phenolphthalein.

and erythema multiforme. This pattern may be due to nalidixic acid (Fig. 10.8).

Toxic epidermal necrolysis   This causes large areas of skin to peel, leaving an underlying erythema and sometimes flaccid bullae. The patients are very ill with fever and malaise, and one-third die, often from bronchopneumonia. Any skin area may be involved, including mucous membranes, so that fluid and electrolyte balance is upset. Apart from cases apparently precipitated by staphylococcal infection (see Ch. 1), drugs producing it include pyrazolones, sulphonamides, hydantoin derivatives and barbiturates (Fig. 10.9).

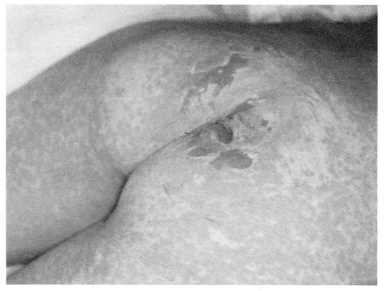

Fig. 10.9   Toxic epidermal necrolysis following barbiturates.

Management

Accurate diagnosis is an important part of therapy.

The drug should be stopped as soon as an adverse reaction is suspected.

Cross-sensitivity of salicylates with food preservatives can be a problem and may be impossible to prove.

It may be dangerous to re-administer a suspected drug: a suitable alternative is almost always available. Patch testing for contact eczema and prick testing for urticaria may help.

In vitro tests such as lymphocyte transformation, macrophage inhibition and basophil degranulation are experimental and costly. Calamine preparations and mild topical steroids, with oral antihistamines are the mainstay of management. The more severe reactions such as erythema multiforme, lupus erythematosus, severe purpura, exfoliative erythroderma and toxic epidermal necrolysis may require hospitalization and systemic steroids.

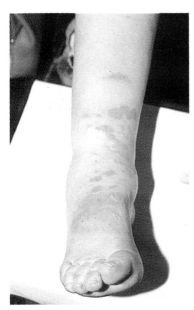

Fig. 10.8   A vesico-bullous rash due to nalidixic acid.

FURTHER READING

Bruinsma W 1982 The file of adverse reactions to the skin. In: A guide to drug eruptions, Zwaluw, De

Pillsbury D, Heaton C 1980 Manual of Dermatology, W B Saunders, Philadelphia

Rook A, Wilkinson D S, Ebling F J G 1979 Textbook of Dermatology. Blackwell Scientific Publications, Oxford

P. Hall-Smith

11. Lichen Planus and Pityriasis Rosea

LICHEN PLANUS

Lichen Planus accounts for about 1% of all dermatological consultations. It is usually seen in adult life and its distribution is worldwide. The aetiology is obscure but there are suggestions that antigenic stimulation results in an immunological reaction in the skin.

Viral and bacterial antigens may be involved and histocompatibility antigens 3 and 5 appear frequently in lichen planus. Many transplant patients develop lichen planus-like oral eruptions. Lichen planus and primary biliary cirrhosis are often associated, the latter being similar to chronic graft-versus-host disease. It may also be associated with chronic hepatitis; oral lesions are especially common in these patients.

Clinical features The onset of the disease is usually slow, though occasional cases may show a generalized rash within a few days. The primary and characteristic lesion is the papule which is polygonal or multiangular in shape, flat-topped and shiny. This may be punctate, 1–2 mm in diameter,

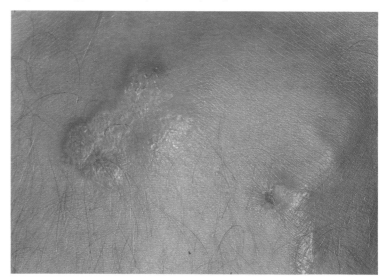

Fig. 11.1 Hypertrophic lichen planus showing Wickam's striae.

occasionally much larger, and an aggregate of these papules can give rise to a large plaque. With the aid of a hand lens, Wickham's striae (Fig. 11.1), white dots and fine white lines, can be seen on the surface of the papules which in the early stages are pink in colour. Later the lesions become violaceous and pigmented.

The most common sites of early lesions are the flexor aspects of the wrist and lumbar region, although lesions may occur on any part of the body. Annular lesions are not uncommon (Fig. 11.2) and are often seen on the glans penis; thicker, hypertrophic (Fig. 11.1) lesions occur on the legs.

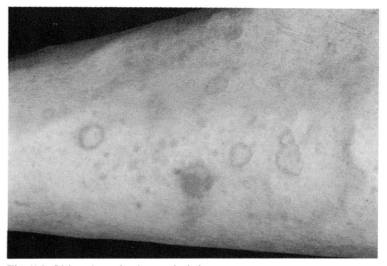

Fig. 11.2   Lichen planus showing annular lesions.

The Koebner phenomenon (Fig. 11.3), a sign of active lichen planus, is a line of papules at a site of trauma. In the buccal mucosa (Fig. 11.4), there is a reticulate pattern or white lines of white plaques—the latter especially on the tongue. Other affected mucosal surfaces are the lips, vagina, anus and stomach. Nails and scalp are less often involved.

Drugs may give rise to a lichen planus-like eruption (lichenoid). Mepacrine is the best documented offender; heavy metals, antidiabetic drugs, phenothiazines, beta-blockers, quinidine, thiazides, penicillamine, naproxen and antituberculous drugs have all been incriminated.

Management   Most minor and non-erosive cases clear without treatment within 6–18 months and assurance of this is all that is needed in the majority. Treatment is largely symptomatic. The itching lessens and the individual lesions become flatter and darker in colour. This post-inflammatory hyperpigmentation usually clears though it may take many months. A minority of patients have second attacks.

Topical steroid creams and ointments allay the itch and possibly aid spontaneous resolution. Betamethasone valerate cream or ointment or the more potent clobetasol propionate should be rubbed in twice daily to itchy, infiltrated lesions over relatively localized areas. Hypertrophic

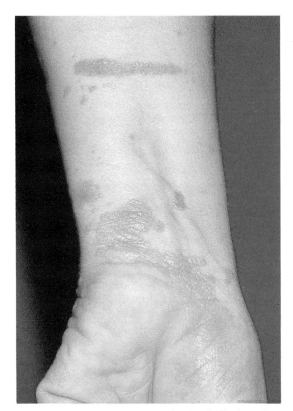

Fig. 11.3 Coalescent lichen planus showing the Koebner phenomenon.

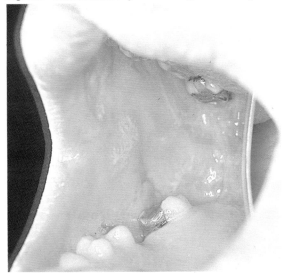

Fig. 11.4 Lichen planus of the buccal mucosa.

lesions, usually on the legs, may be treated with the same topical steroids
under polythene occlusion or by intralesional injection of triamcinolone.
Medicated occlusive bandaging (Zinc Paste and Coal Tar Bandage or
Zinc Paste and Ichthammol Bandage) is useful when the patient cannot

stop scratching. With widespread lesions and mild discomfort, calamine lotion with 1% phenol, aqueous cream with 0.5% phenol and 0.5% menthol or betamethasone valerate cream 0.025% are appropriate.

There have been reports of the successful use of oral 8-methoxy-psoralen photo-chemotherapy (PUVA). It may be effective against generalized symptomatic lichen planus and maintenance therapy may not be required once it is completely cleared.

The disease responds to systemic corticosteroids and ACTH but they should be reserved for the small number of severe and widespread cases where the itching is intolerable and/or there are severe erosive mucous membrane lesions (Fig. 11.5) and progressive nail destruction (see Ch. 20). The symptoms are relieved and the lesions may clear completely during treatment. Although some relapse may occur when the drug is discontinued, most of the gain is usually held.

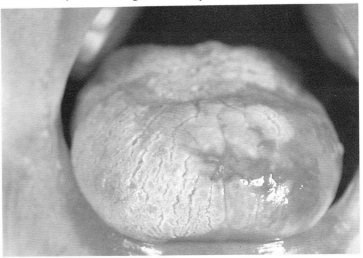

Fig. 11.5 Erosive lichen planus of the tongue.

Prednisolone, or its equivalent, in a dose of 20–30 mg daily with gradual weaning over a period of 4–6 weeks, is an effective regime. In these severe and florid cases, ACTH or tetracosactrin may be preferred.

Metronidazole has been reported as effective in cases of lichen planus where the responsible bacterial antigen was sensitive to it. In some cases there has been dramatic involution of the lesions. Metronidazole is also effective in erosive ulcerative-lichen planus of the oral mucosa in a dose of 250 mg three times daily for 2 weeks. Systemic steroid therapy is needed in unresponsive, painful erosive mucous membrane lesions. Less severe cases may be helped by triamcinolone in a special base (see Ch. 18).

PITYRIASIS ROSEA

The cause of pityriasis rosea is unknown. There is epidemiological evidence of possible infection but no causative organism has been isolated and innoculation experiments have failed to reproduce the disease.

Clinical features   Pityriasis rosea is a self-limiting acute eruption of annulo-squamous discs on the trunk and proximal part of the limbs. It is usually preceded by a 'herald patch' which may appear anywhere on the trunk, the chest being a frequent site. This is an erythematous disc 1–5 cm in diameter. After 7 or 10 days, small satellite lesions appear. These enlarge and other discoid lesions suddenly appear, covering most of the trunk (Fig. 11.6). The neck and peripheral areas are rarely involved.

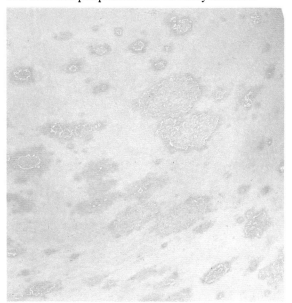

Fig. 11.6 Pityriasis rosea showing a 'herald patch'.

The pink, scaly lesions are often oval and lie parallel to the skin creases (Fig. 11.7). Scaling begins in the centre of these discs, which drop off leaving a characteristic collarette of scales around the periphery. When the lesions begin to fade on the trunk others may still appear on the limbs; severe cases affect the hands and feet. The total duration is usually 6–8 weeks but, occasionally, it persists for 3 months or longer. Pruritus may be minimal or severe. It is uncommon after the age of 35.

The differential diagnosis includes discoid seborrhoeic eczema, psoriasis, parapsoriasis, ringworm and secondary syphilis. Drugs for rheumatoid arthritis, gold, d-penicillamine and levamisole, have been reported as giving a pityriasis rosea-like rash.

Management   Spontaneous resolution is the rule, although scratching and secondary eczema may delay healing. Asymptomatic cases need no treatment.

Troublesome itching may respond to simple emollients such as aqueous cream or oily calamine lotion. If they do not control itch then betamethasone valerate cream as a short-term measure should be effective. Emulsifying ointment can be used as a soap substitute or one of

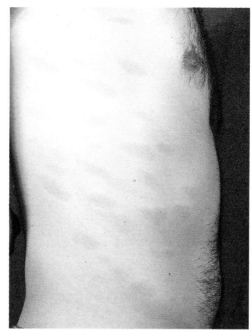

Fig. 11.7 Pityriasis rosea showing lesions parallel to the skin creases.

the proprietary emollient bath additives will relieve skin dryness and pruritus.

Sunlight or artificial ultra-violet light is believed to alleviate the symptoms and alter the course of the disease. Consecutive daily erythemogenic exposures for 5–7 days can result in a substantial reduction in pruritus and in the extent of the disease in an appreciable number of patients. Therapy seems to be most beneficial to patients receiving it within the first week.

FURTHER READING

Arndt K A, Paul B S, Stern R S, Parrish J A 1983 Treatment of pityriasis rosea with U.V. radiation. Archives of Dermatology 119: 381

Gonzalez E, Momtaz T K, Freedman S 1984 Bilateral comparison of generalized lichen planus treated with psoralens and ultra-violet A. Journal of the American Academy of Dermatology 10: 958–961

Graham-Brown R A, Sarkany I, Sherlock S 1982 Lichen planus and primary biliary cirrhosis. British Journal of Dermatology 106: 699–703

Hall-Smith P, Cairns R J 1981 Dermatology: current concepts and practice. Butterworth, London, p 60–61

Messenger A G, Knox E G, Summerly R, Muston H L, Ilderton E 1982 Case clustering in pityriasis rosea; support for role of an infective agent. British Medical Journal 284: 371

Ortonne J P, Thivolet J, Sannwald C 1978 Oral photochemotherapy in the treatment of lichen planus. British Journal of Dermatology 99: 77

Samman P D 1979 Lichen planus and lichenoid eruptions. In: Rook A, Wilkinson D S, Ebling F J G (eds) Textbook of dermatology. Blackwell Scientific Publications, Oxford

Shelley W B, Shelley E D 1984 Urinary tract infection as a cause of lichen planus; metronidazole therapy. Journal of the American Academy of Dermatology 10: suppl. 5, pt. 2, 905

12. Skin Manifestations of Systemic Disease and Anogenital Pruritus

SKIN MANIFESTATIONS OF SYSTEMIC DISEASE

Many systemic diseases are reflected on the skin and a knowledge of the presentation can often aid in the identification of a possible underlying cause.

Dry Skin (Xerosis)

Clinical features Dry skin is particularly common in the elderly. It often itches and in many patients who itch with no definite rash, the cause is dry skin. However, it may be the presenting feature of hypothyroidism and be linked with sarcoidosis, lymphoma and essential fatty acid deficiency. Its recent onset should alert the doctor to a possible underlying cause.

Management Management is with topical applications including emollients and urea-containing creams to enhance skin hydration.

Itching

Clinical features Systemic causes of pruritus include drugs, biliary obstruction, connective tissue disorders, chronic renal failure (Fig. 12.1), pregnancy, blood disorders (such as iron deficiency), lymphomas, internal carcinoma, hypothyroidism, thyrotoxicosis, malabsorption, psychogenic and neurological disease and parasitic infestations; the symptom merits thorough investigation.

Management Symptomatic treatment involves oral antihistamines but itching due to systemic disease responds poorly. Light clothing is useful and calamine lotion or menthol 1% in an aqueous cream helps. Topical anaesthetic or antihistamine creams or ointments carry a real risk of sensitization and are contraindicated.

Cholestyramine is used in pruritus due to cholestasis. Dialysis, low protein diet and subtotal parathyroidectomy may be indicated in some patients with uraemic pruritus.

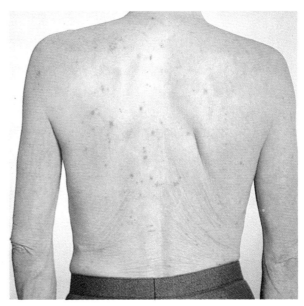

Fig. 12.1   Excoriations are visible in this patient with itching associated with chronic renal failure.

Urticaria (see Ch. 4)

Management   Foods, drugs and inhalants should be looked for in acute cases but in 40% or more of these no cause is found. In chronic urticaria (lasting longer than 6 weeks), which is more common in middle-aged women, usually no cause is found but the psyche is often important. Most cases of chronic urticaria have a good prognosis. Treatment consists of removing the cause, if possible, and use of antihistamines of the H_1 blocking type.

Alopecia (see Ch. 20)

Systemic causes of scalp hair fall include drugs, some of which—such as cytotoxic drugs and anticoagulants—have a toxic effect on growing hair. This is reversible. Some disorders associated with severe physical or mental stress may precipitate telogen and thus cause hair fall a few months later; they include fever, surgery, active colitis, meningitis, schizophrenia and pregnancy. Hypo- and hyper-thyroidism, iron deficiency and systemic lupus erythematosus are also causes of hair fall.

Purpura

Purpura may be thrombocytopenic or non-thrombocytopenic. Palpable lesions mean that an allergic vasculitis (Fig. 12.2) is probable which may be drug-induced.

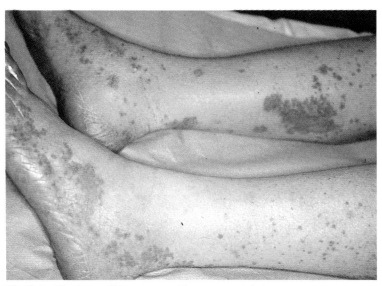

Fig. 12.2 Allergic vasculitis—purpura with some necrotic lesions.

Management   Management is by bed rest and below-knee support bandages when mobile are useful.

Thrombocytopenic purpura may be idiopathic or drug-induced. Treatment of acute attacks is by fresh blood transfusion and corticosteroids.

Scurvy is still seen, particularly in people living alone and lacking vitamin C in the diet. Lower limb bruises should alert doctors to it (Fig. 12.3) and prescription of ascorbic acid and attention to diet is imperative in its management.

Toxic epidermal necrolysis (TEN) and staphylococcal scalded skin syndrome (SSSS) (see Chs. 1 & 10)

Pyoderma gangrenosum

Clinical features   Fully developed, this is a deep ulcer with an advancing undermined border and an adherent necrotic and pustular centre. Lesions are usually single over the shin but may be multiple and can occur anywhere. They may start as pustules and become plaques which ulcerate. Causes include ulcerative colitis, Crohn's disease, paraproteinaemia and myeloma, and both rheumatoid-like and rheumatoid arthritis.

Management   This includes application of topical antiseptics, intralesional steroids injected at the borders of lesions, oral sulphasalazine or clofazamine, systemic corticosteroids, ACTH or long acting tetracosactrin.

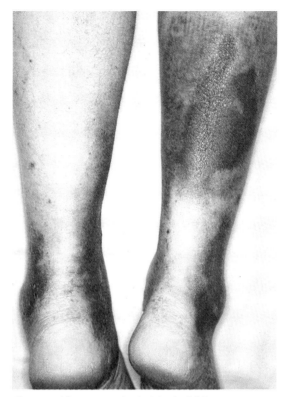

Fig. 12.3 Scurvy—extensive bruising is visible.

Necrobiosis lipoidica

Clinical features   These yellow-brown plaques are seen particularly over the shins,
characteristically in diabetes mellitus. In fact, two-thirds of patients with
necrobiosis lipoidica will be found to be diabetic and others will become
diabetic later. Chronic lesions are associated with atrophic skin, which
may ulcerate.

Management   Early lesions can be aborted by intralesional corticosteroid injection, but
injection of well-established lesions will produce ulcers. Chronic lesions
may merit cosmetic cover.

Xanthomatosis

Clinical features   Associated with hyperlipidaemia, this may be primary and inherited
(Fig. 12.4). In 10−20% of patients it is secondary to conditions such as
alcohol over-indulgence, diabetes mellitus, hypothyroidism and
cholestasis. Primary and secondary hyperlipidaemia may co-exist.
Thorough investigation, including electrophoresis and family history, is
very important.

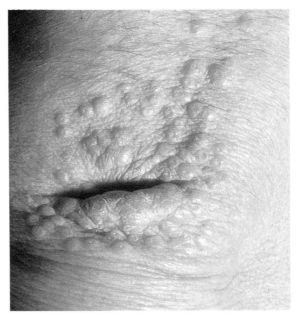

Fig. 12.4 Multiple xanthomata with lipid deposits over elbow.

Management Management, which will include lipid-lowering agents when indicated, causes exanthamata to disappear. The development of plaques on the eyelids (xanthelasma) may need local treatment by cauterization or careful painting with trichloroacetic acid.

Crohn's disease and ulcerative colitis

Skin lesions, apart from those in the mouth and perianal region, affect 10–15% of patients with Crohn's disease. They include erythema nodosum, a hypersensitivity vasculitis, in 4–7%, and pyoderma gangrenosum in less than 2%. However, perianal inflammation may be the first sign of the bowel disorder. Anal and perianal erythema and oedema and tense oedematous cyanotic skin tags at the anal margin are important signs.

The incidence of skin lesions in ulcerative colitis, excluding perianal and mouth lesions, is 10%: 4% have erythema nodosum and 2% pyoderma gangrenosum. Erythema nodosum is closely related to the activity of the bowel disease but pyoderma gangrenosum may precede, accompany or follow an episode of bowel inflammation.

Aphthous ulceration in the mouth occurs in about 20% of patients with Crohn's disease and 10% of those with ulcerative colitis. Such ulceration is common with other extra-intestinal manifestations of Crohn's disease. Occasionally Crohn's disease involves the buccal mucosa producing swelling and a corrugated appearance (Fig. 12.5).

Treatment of the bowel disease is paramount.

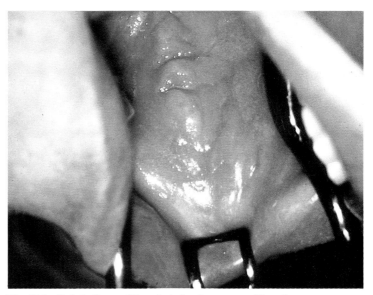

Fig. 12.5 Crohn's disease of the mouth showing corrugated buccal mucosa.

Blistering disorders (see Ch. 18)

Connective tissue disorders

In many of these, management is often principally of the primary condition.

Systemic sclerosis The first skin changes are usually those of Raynaud's syndrome and the hands must be kept warm. Gastrointestinal, respiratory and renal function must be investigated. Topical antiseptic preparations for complications of Raynaud's syndrome, such as fingertip ulceration, may help.

Systemic lupus erythematosus (SLE) In its most benign form localized to the skin, lupus presents as disc-shaped cutaneous lesions. There are no signs and symptoms of systemic disease and there is no serological evidence of systemic disease. However, skin lesions are initially present in 25% of patients with SLE. In the course of their disease, 80% of SLE patients have skin lesions: they may be discoid.

Management of the many types of SLE skin lesions involves treating the primary condition which includes oral corticosteroids, cytotoxic drugs and antimalarials. Potent topical corticosteroids are helpful in some instances.

Dermatomyositis It may present with violaceous erythema over the face and the backs of the fingers and/or pectoral and pelvic girdle muscle weakness. A primary malignant cause is found in about 15% of adults and this should if possible be treated.

Systemic corticosteroids, such as prednisolone, are needed for the management of this condition although any underlying malignancy must be excluded in patients over 40 years of age.

Polyarteritis nodosa   Skin lesions in this systemic disease are non-specific, including purpura and urticaria, and management is of the primary condition.

Porphyrias

Porphyria cutanea tarda

Clinical features   Skin fragility, blisters, hypertrichosis, hyperpigmentation and onycholysis are the features of this disease. Lesions are predominantly on light-exposed areas. The middle-aged are particularly affected.

Management   Management includes elimination of alcohol, oestrogen or iron ingestion and avoidance of environmental toxins which may have triggered the disease. Regular phlebotomy remains the treatment of choice.

Erythropoietic protoporphyria

Clinical features   This autosomal dominant dermatosis usually presents in the summer with burning of exposed skin. It generally begins by the age of 2 years. Blisters, erythema, purpura, swelling and characteristic linear scars appear, particularly on the backs of hands and the middle third of the face.

Management   Treatment is with suitable sunblockers of long-wave UV light and oral beta-carotene is indicated.

Sarcoidosis

Clinical features   This condition produces non-caseating granulomata, commonly in lymph nodes, lungs, skin and eyes. Specific granulomatous skin lesions may be macules, papules, nodules or plaques. The most common non-specific lesion is erythema nodosum.

Management   Acute sarcoidosis, with erythema nodosum and bilateral hilar adenopathy, is usually self-limiting and needs no specific therapy. Intralesional steroids may help chronic cutaneous lesions, particularly plaques.

Cutaneous T-cell lymphomas

Clinical features   This term covers several malignant skin diseases of unknown cause including mycosis fungoides (MF). MF has three stages: (1) premycotic non-specific eczematous, (2) plaque, (3) tumour. Pruritus is variable. The first stage may last less than a year or for 30 years or more.

Erythroderma can develop at any stage and may be exfoliative. Lymph nodes become palpable at any time in MF but particularly in the tumour stage. There may not be frank lymphoma on histology. Death in MF is usually secondary to infection.

Management   This includes, at different stages, topical corticosteroids, topical nitrogen mustard, ionizing radiation—particularly as high energy electrons—PUVA and systemic chemotherapy.

ANOGENITAL PRURITUS

Pruritus ani

Clinical features   Pruritus ani is more common in men. It may be primary or be secondary to local or systemic causes. Causes include poor hygiene, eczema, psoriasis, intertrigo, candidosis (sometimes associated with diabetes mellitus), ringworm, viral warts, threadworms (Fig. 12.6), diarrhoea, excessive hair; there are many others.

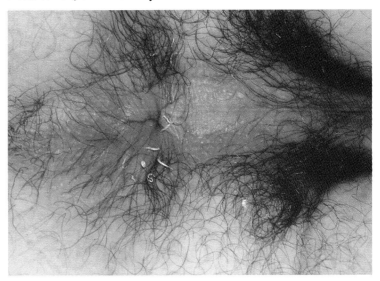

Fig. 12.6   Threadworms are visible at the anal orifice.

Management   Anal hygiene is important. Underclothes must be changed often because soiled underpants and faecal skin contamination combine to irritate the skin. Straining on defaecation should be avoided. The patient should sit for 3−4 minutes on the toilet after defaecation before gently wiping the anal region clean. Soft toilet paper should be used. Dampening it helps. Aggressive wiping produces further trauma. Cotton, loose-fitting underpants are preferred to occlusive trunks.

For patients who cannot stop rubbing, doing it next to the itchy area often gives some relief.

An aqueous solution of silver nitrate (1/6−1/4%) applied to the clean anal area and allowed to dry is followed by 1% hydrocortisone cream; twice daily or after bowel movements. St Mark's lotion is a useful alternative (see Formulary).

A warm bath containing 1−2 teaspoonfuls of ordinary table or cooking salt is also soothing. Oral antihistamines, particularly hydroxyzine, can help.

Antifungal or other medication should be prescribed if needed. Threadworms should be treated with antihelminthics and hygienic measures. The whole family must be treated.

Surgery is sometimes the answer in some specific conditions, e.g. anal fissure or haemorrhoids.

Scrotal irritation

Clinical features Occasional patients complain of one or more of the following related to the scrotal skin—redness, pruritus, discomfort, burning—and yet there is nothing abnormal on repeated examination.

Management Management of these possibly neurotic or psychotic patients demands understanding and patience from the doctor.

Pruritus vulvae

Clinical features This may be an extension of pruritus ani but it has many and varied causes, both cutaneous and systemic. Cutaneous causes include contact dermatitis (sometimes due to application of medicaments), constitutional eczema, psoriasis, scabies, lichen planus and lichen sclerosus et atrophicus (white spot disease). In the last, seen particularly in postmenopausal women but sometimes before puberty, atrophic skin— sometimes with blisters—occurs in discrete lesions which later become confluent. It forms a 'figure of eight' pattern around the vulva and perianal region.

Itching may be precipitated by a vaginal discharge, the cause of which must be found. In diabetics it is usually due to vulval cutaneous candidosis. The psyche can be important in chronic pruritus vulvae. Time should be spent discussing the chronic symptoms with the patient.

Management In general, topical steroid creams are useful but pruritus vulvae should be appropriately investigated.

J-H. Saurat

13. Paediatric Dermatology

Most skin diseases occurring in childhood have their counterparts in adults and their management is covered elsewhere. The following are reviewed:

1. The important characteristics of the child's skin relevant to treatment
2. The modern management of some skin diseases occurring in childhood
3. The topically applied medications potentially dangerous in children.

THE CHILD'S SKIN: CHARACTERISTICS RELEVANT TO THERAPY

Child's skin as a barrier

The barrier function is one of the most important properties of the skin. It prevents water loss and modulates the penetration of foreign substances.

Stratum corneum function in infants

Percutaneous absorption involves slow diffusion (not active transport) through the stratum corneum. The stratum corneum of mature neonates is an efficient barrier. This is not so, however, in preterm infants or those with diseased skin in whom skin permeability is increased.

The crucial difference in percutaneous absorption between adults and infants is primarily due to the ratio of surface area to body weight. The systemic level of a drug delivered by percutaneous absorption in infants may be as high as 2.7 times that in an adult, increasing the risk of toxicity. Occlusion may dramatically enhance percutaneous absorption. The napkin area in infants and babies is permanently under occlusion and this should be considered when treating it.

Likewise in infants, water loss from the skin is considerable from transepidermal water loss (TEWL) and eccrine sweating. TEWL is increased in preterm infants, in infants with diseased skin and low environmental humidity; excessive water loss may even lead to hypernatraemic dehydration.

Infant cutaneous appendages

Sweat glands The sweat glands are already mature and functional in neonates and infants but the neurological control of sweating is immature. A poor sweating response may therefore be expected in neonates and especially in preterm infants, even leading to fever in a hot environment.

Sebaceous glands The sebaceous glands function from the 17th week of gestation. Sebum production, however, decreases in the early weeks after birth when maternal hormonal influence ceases. In neonates the skin surface lipids are mainly sebum, the chemical composition of which is very similar to that of the adult.

Two periods in childhood are related both to sebum secretion and skin care. The first is the seborrhoeic period, the duration of which varies from baby to baby. This is the period of neonatal acne and of so-called 'seborrheic dermatitis' (see p. 113). The second period is later on in childhood, when loss of sebum secretion leads to inadequate skin lubrication, excess dryness and increased susceptibility to chapping, especially during the winter. Lack of sebum secretion on the scalp in prepubertal children may contribute to their increased incidence of tinea capitis.

MODERN MANAGEMENT OF SOME CHILDHOOD DISEASES

Napkin area eruptions

Clinical features Napkin rash is not specific but a reaction in a localized area in the microclimate produced by plastic or rubber napkin cover occlusion, and prolonged contact with urine and faeces. This promotes inflammation and may lead to *Candida albicans* superinfection in the infant with oral candidosis. It is important to define the part of the perineal skin primarily involved.

Intertrigo (folds involved) This may be due to a number of factors: heat: moisture and sweat retention together cause maceration; bacteria proliferate and contribute to its perpetuation. The skin becomes erythematous and the lesions may erode.

Intertrigo in the genitocrural folds may be a sign of seborrhoeic dermatitis often accompanied by involvement of the axillae, neck folds, retro-auricular area, umbilicus and scalp ('scaly cradle cap') (Fig. 13.1). Its cause is poorly understood. Some believe seborrhoeic dermatitis to be a variant of atopic dermatitis. Simple maceration and seborrhoeic dermatitis are often complicated by candidosis. This produces satellite pustular lesions with peripheral scaling (Fig. 13.2). When there is only a perineal dermatitis with satellite pustules, the probable diagnosis is a primary candidosis. Primary perineal candidosis complicates intestinal infection, oral thrush and the use of some oral antibiotics, e.g. ampicillin.

Psoriasiform lesions may start in the folds and spread to the whole

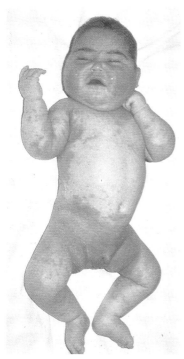

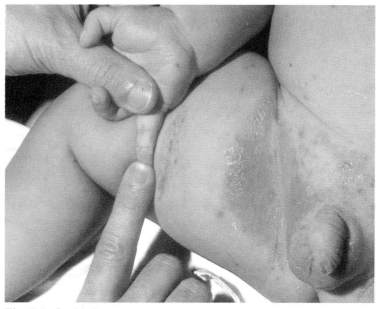

Fig. 13.2 Candidosis.

Fig. 13.1 Seborrhoeic dermatitis treated for weeks with a strong topical steroid. Note the persistence of the erythema and the cushingoid appearance of the child. (Courtesy of J M Bonnetblanc, MD.)

perineal area, lower abdomen and thighs. Whether or not this 'napkin psoriasis' represents an initial attack of psoriasis is controversial but candidosis probably plays a part. In any patient only long-term observation and the appearance of more classical lesions of psoriasis elsewhere will provide the answer.

Convex surfaces involved
Folds spared

When parchment-like erythema similar to a scald occurs on convex surfaces (convexities of the buttocks, the thighs, scrotum and pubis), sparing the folds, the likely cause of the napkin eruption is primary irritant dermatitis (Fig. 13.3). This is readily infected with bacteria to produce pustules, erosions and nodules.

Granuloma gluteale infantum presents the appearance of multiple-acquired angiomata. Well-demarcated nodules, sometimes as large as a cherry, appear in the perineal area. Their cause is not clear. Some but not all patients have been exposed to prolonged application of potent corticosteroids.

Ammonia was widely believed to play an important role in napkin dermatitis; it arises from the action of *Brevibacterium ammoniagenes* in the faeces or urine. As a unique primary causative agent of napkin rash, it has been challenged. In fact, the dermatitis results from long contact of urine and faeces with the perineal skin under airtight occlusion. Occasionally it is localized at the margins of the napkin.

Folds and convex surfaces involved

When maceration, candidosis, bacterial superinfection and prolonged contact with urine and faeces are all present, the whole perineal skin and buttocks may be involved.

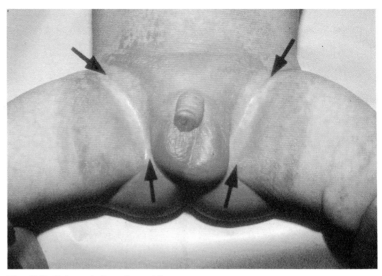

Fig. 13.3   Primary irritant dermatitis.

Management   When there are pustular lesions, *Candida albicans* may be seen and cultured. The basis of all treatment is to remove the contactants (urine, faeces, napkins) from the skin and eliminate maceration by keeping it dry. Plastic and rubber pants should be avoided and frequent napkin changes prescribed.

The skin should be gently rinsed with tepid water several times a day to remove urine and faeces; imidazole lotions several times a day are helpful. Water repellant barrier creams and simple covering agents such as Zinc and Castor Oil Cream may be helpful.

Other eruptions of the napkin area   Impetigo (see Ch. 1), atopic dermatitis (see Ch. 7) and histiocytosis X can localize in the napkin area.

Ichthyoses

Clinical features   The hereditary ichthyoses are characterized by the accumulation of visible scales on the skin. The four principal types differ in their clinical presentation, genetics, histopathology and pathogenesis. Each affected child should be evaluated carefully, to characterize the specific type, on which depends the prognosis, pathological associations, therapy and genetic counselling.

Ichthyosis vulgaris, the commonest form, is a dominant disease which spares flexures. Recessive X-linked ichthyosis (RXLI) is the second most common form and may involve the flexures. The basic abnormality is a deficiency of steroid sulphatase in skin and other tissues. This leads to inability to remove sulphate from cholesterol sulphate and other steroids. Accumulation of cholesterol sulphate in the stratum corneum is thought to alter normal desquamation. Lamellar ichthyosis (non-bullous congenital ichthyosiform erythroderma) is one of the most severe forms.

The whole skin is involved and ectropion is common. A bullous type of ichthyosiform erythroderma exists.

Management

Management consists of adding emollients to the bathwater and the frequent application of emollients to the skin. Vitamin A acid ointment 0.1% should be tried, as should salicylic acid, 1–3% in soft paraffin, and urea.

Three recent major breakthroughs have modified the management of some ichthyoses: (1) the discovery of the enzyme abnormality in recessive X-linked ichthyosis, (2) treatment with synthetic retinoids, (3) prenatal diagnosis by in utero-fetal skin biopsy (also applicable to epidermolysis bullosa).

A good response has been reported to topical application of cholesterol in X-linked ichthyosis.

Retinoids in childhood

Severe psoriasis and hereditary defects of keratinization (e.g. some ichthyoses) are the best indications for synthetic retinoid therapy in childhood.

Clinical similarities between the skin changes of hypovitaminosis A and certain changes in keratinization provided the rationale for first testing of vitamin A treatment. Natural vitamin A, however, is severely toxic at the doses needed for the control of keratinization diseases. Synthetic vitamin A analogues which are more active and better tolerated than the parent compound have been developed; two of these retinoids, isotretinoin and etretinate are available. Already two important facts about their use in ichthyosis are apparent:

1. Etretinate is the drug of choice over isotretinoin
Etretinate has already been used for long periods (up to 6 years with daily doses of 0.5–1 mg/kg/body weight) in children, including the very young (less than 1 year of age) with no serious side-effects. In contrast, children treated with isotretinoin developed severe skeletal problems (premature partial epiphyseal closure, hyperostosis). Whether this is due to the higher doses of isotretinoin needed to control the ichthyosis (up to 2–3 mg/kg/day) or to distinct pharmacological properties is unknown.

2. All the ichthyoses are not equally responsive to retinoids
Lammellar ichthyosis is dramatically improved by etretinate. It must be given continuously at the lowest dose necessary for controlling scaling (usually 0.25 to 0.5 mg/kg/day). No serious side-effects have yet been observed; growth and development are not hampered by long-term etretinate treatment.

The low morbidity of RXLI seldom justifies etretinate therapy in childhood. Ichthyosis vulgaris may be exacerbated by etretinate. In bullous congenital ichthyosiform erythroderma (epidermolytic hyperkeratosis), the hyperkeratotic lesions decrease during treatment but are replaced by areas of bullae and denudation so that patient compliance is poor.

Epidermolysis bullosa

Clinical features   The inherited disorder of epidermolysis bullosa is characterized by skin blistering after minor trauma. The severity ranges from occasional mild blistering of hands and feet to severe widespread bulla formation with non-healing erosions, infections and disabling scarring (Fig. 13.4). There are several forms of epidermolysis bullosa.

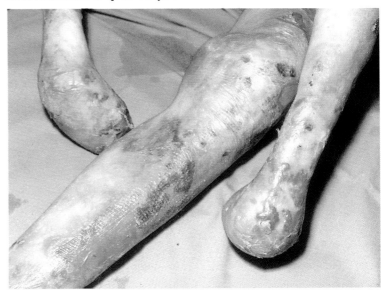

Fig. 13.4 Epidermolysis bullosa.

Management   Morphological and biochemical studies have greatly increased our understanding of several of these diseases yet therapy remains largely supportive. Phenytoin may help some patients with the dystrophic forms by reducing dermal collagenase which is thought to play a major part in the pathogenesis. Prenatal diagnosis of the severe forms of epidermolysis bullosa is now possible; foetoscopy and foetal skin sampling offer early detection in families already stricken with one such child.

Viral exanthamata

Clinical features   These occur especially in childhood. Acute eruptive papulo vesicular and urticarial and eczematous eruptions occur following Coxsackie virus or adenovirus infection. This diagnosis should be considered in a child with a bizarre atypical rash and with a history of recent respiratory tract or gastrointestinal infection.

Management   This is conservative. If pruritus is severe, Calamine Lotion may be applied or systemic antihistamines given.

TOPICAL DRUGS WITH POTENTIALLY HARMFUL SYSTEMIC EFFECTS IN INFANCY

Systemic side-effects of topical therapy in infancy may cause concern. Several specific factors in infancy may lead to systemic side-effects: (1) the alteration of percutaneous absorption and the ratio of surface area to body weight (see p. 111), (2) immature metabolism of and response to drugs, (3) the occlusive effect of napkins.

The risk is greater when the drug is applied to diseased skin in which percutaneous absorption is increased (Table 13.1). A number of topical drugs are potentially harmful in infancy (Table 13.2); they must either be avoided or used with caution. Only drugs still currently used in paediatric dermatology are detailed below.

Table 13.1 Disorders associated with increased risk of adverse systemic reactions to topical drugs

Burns
Epidermolysis bullosa
Ichthyosis
Infantile atopic dermatitis
Seborrhoeic dermatitis
Napkin dermatitis
Psoriasis
Ulcers

Table 13.2 Some topical drugs with potentially harmful systemic effects in infancy

	Drug	Systemic risk
Drugs to be avoided	Boric acid, borate	Shock, renal failure, death
	Phenol	Methaemoglobinaemia convulsions
	Mercury	Acrodynia, nephropathy
	Hexachlorophene	Vacuolization of myelin
	Podophyllin	Neuropathy
Drugs to be avoided or to be used with caution	Iodine	Hypothyroidism
	Camphor	Convulsions
	Silver nitrate	Methaemoglobinaemia
	Trichlorocarban	Methaemoglobinaemia
	Neomycin	Deafness
	Lindane	Convulsions
	Benzyl benzonate	Not well documented
	Salicylic acid	Acidosis, coma
	Coal tar	Methaemoglobinaemia
	Steroids	Similar to systemic use

Salicylic acid

Salicylic acid is used as a keratolytic ('scale remover'). Excessive percutaneous absorption induces acidosis, deep and rapid breathing, convulsions, coma and even death. Children most at risk are those with extensive seborrhoeic dermatitis, psoriasis or ichthyosis, treated with high concentrations of salicylic acid ointment several times a day on large surface areas. Salicylic acid has no ill-effect if the area of treatment is limited (less than 25% body surface) and the concentration is low (less than 2%).

Iodine

Repeated topical use of iodine in neonates and infants is associated with significant changes in thyroid function (goitre and hypothyroidism). Absorption of iodine occurs in neonates treated with povidone iodine but without altering thyroid function.

Lindane and other topical treatments of scabies

The safety of gamma benzene hexachloride (Lindane) has been the subject of considerable controversy. Massive contamination, e.g. by accidental ingestion, produces nausea, vomiting, headache, apnoea and even death. Repeated applications over long periods may produce these major side-effects.

Even a single application of 1% Lindane may be toxic in infants and signs of toxicity such as hypotonia, apathy and irritability may go unrecognised. Despite controversial reports there are still no scientifically proven guidelines for Lindane use in infants and young children concerning (1) the concentration (1% or less?), (2) the need for a hot, soapy bath before its application, (3) the shortest time of application needed to cure scabies (8–12 hours are recommended and repeated use is strongly discouraged), (4) the usefulness of washing after application to prevent further absorption. Alternative scabicides exist although they are not necessarily safer. Crotamiton 10% is less active than Lindane but appears safer, despite a case of methaemoglobinemia in a 2-month-old baby. Benzyl benzonate is as effective as Lindane but does not appear safer.

A premature, malnourished infant was poisoned after one application of 1% Lindane, with a blood level 17 times greater than expected. Decreased subcutaneous fat tissue may have caused the preferential redistribution of the highly lipid-soluble Lindane into the infant brain.

Topical corticosteroids

Adverse systemic effects from topical corticosteroids applied to the skin, used at inappropriate potency and for prolonged periods, include Cushing's syndrome, growth retardation or cessation and intra-cranial hypertension. After warnings of the adverse effects of potent topical steroids, some paediatricians seek safety in such low concentrations of weak steroids that the ultimate dose seems homeopathic. The choice in children with problems such as severe atopic dermatitis is either a low-potency steroid, the clinical effect of which will be poor, or medium- to high-potency steroid to control the eczema quickly. A rapid and marked therapeutic effect can be obtained with potent steroids, even applied only once daily, but this is often accompanied by a fall in plasma cortisol (Table 13.3). Physicians not experienced in using topical steroids should avoid them rather than expose a child to undesirable effects (by choosing a strong steroid) or let the dermatosis perpetuate unabated (by choosing ineffective doses of weak steroids). Topical steroids should be used with care on the face and the napkin area; some prefer to avoid them at these sites.

Table 13.3 Correlation between clinical improvement and decrease in plasma cortisol in children with atopic dermatitis

Topical steroid	Clinical improvement % of initial values Clinical score, day 6	Plasma cortisol % of initial values
Betamethasone diproprionate	66	39
Diflucortolone valerate	40	27
Halcinonide	32	61
Clobetasone butyrate	37	79
Desonide	38	100
Fluocortin butyl ester	23	100

The greater clinical improvement corresponds to the greater decrease in plasma cortisol (adapted from Queille, Pommarede and Saurat, 1984)

FURTHER READING

Cooper T W, Bauer E A 1984 Epidermolysis bullosa: a review. Pediatric Dermatology 1: 181
Hardy J D, Davison S H, Higgins M U 1973 Sweat tests in the newborn period. Archives of Disease in Childhood 48: 316–18
Leyden J J, Katz S, Stewart R, Kligman A 1977 Urinary ammonia and ammonia-producing microorganisms in infants with and without diaper dermatitis. Archives of Dermatology 113: 1678–1680
Queille C, Pommarede R, Saurat J H 1984 Efficacy versus systemic effects of six topical steroids in the treatment of atopic dermatitis of childhood. Pediatric Dermatology 1: 246–53
Rasmussen J E 1979 Percutaneous absorption in children. In: Dobson R L (ed) Year Book of Dermatology. Year Book Medical Publishers, Chicago, p. 15–38
Rasmussen J E 1981 The problem of lindane. Journal of the American Academy of Dermatology 5: 507
Saurat J H 1982 Risques systémiques des médicaments topiques chez l'enfant. Annales de Pediatrie 29: 8–14
van der Schroeff J G, van der Rhee H J 1984 The treatment of children with etretinate. In: Cunliffe W J, Miller A J (eds) Retinoid Therapy, MTP Press Lancaster, p. 39
Williams M L 1983 The ichthyosis—pathogenesis and prenatal diagnosis: a review of recent advances. Pediatric Dermatology 1: 1–24

John H. S. Pettit

14. Tropical Dermatoses

In developing countries poverty and malnutrition are not the only preventable causes of disease. Many infections in these areas have been called 'tropical diseases'. Although some of these (dracunculosis, tinea imbricata, rhinoscleroma etc.) are rarely transported to more temperate areas, others are increasingly being found outside their countries of origin. As most of them are curable, at least in their early stages, a higher index of suspicion will allow them to be recognised before it is too late for effective treatment. In poor areas the cost of treatment may be a major factor to be considered.

ANTHRAX

Man may be affected directly from animals or from animal products, e.g. bone meal or hides.

Clinical features *Cutaneous infection:* in mild cases infection of the skin starts as a raised itchy red nodule, rapidly leading to a central necrotic eschar often wrongly called a malignant pustule. (*B. anthracis* does not cause liquefaction necrosis and pus is never present.) Such cases improve rapidly either alone or with treatment and usually do not leave a scar.

At other times, symptoms start with inflammatory oedema and toxaemia. The initial lesion looks like a severe burn with swelling and redness. It is soon covered with scattered haemorrhagic vesicles which coalesce (Fig. 14.1) and, if left untreated, a deeper eschar is produced leaving a permanent mark on the skin similar to the scar of an oriental sore.

The oedema is often many centimetres thick. It hinders vision if in the upper part of the face and can prevent swallowing or breathing. Many patients have associated toxaemia and reach the doctor in a state of near collapse. Before the emergence of satisfactory treatment some 25% of such cases died.

Pulmonary infection (from spore inhalation) is still often fatal because of the suffocating pulmonary oedema and massive haemorrhagic necrosis of the hilar lymph nodes. Swallowing spores may cause gastro-intestinal

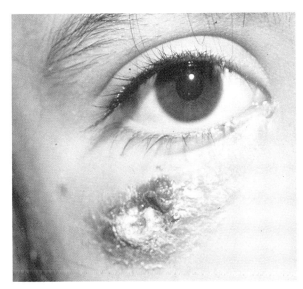

Fig. 14.1 Anthrax.

infection with profuse and bloody diarrhoea. Many less severe cases are probably undiagnosed.

Management

Bacillus anthracis is always susceptible to penicillin; resistance is unknown. In the milder disease nothing more is necessary; intramuscular Procaine Penicillin G, 600 000 units (600 mg) twice daily for a week, may be replaced by oral amoxycillin 250 mg three times a day or ampicillin 500 mg 6-hourly for 10 days. Penicillin-sensitive patients can be given high doses of tetracycline, 500 mg 4-hourly for 10–14 days.

Any of these treatments will eradicate the infective organism but patients may still die if not managed carefully. The greater the oedema, the more problems arise. Associated toxaemia often needs heavy doses of corticosteroids. Considerable loss of circulating fluids into the inflammatory oedema means that suitable steps must be taken to restore the electrolyte balance.

An antitoxin would be most useful in severe cases but none has been developed. A vaccine is available for individuals open to heavy exposure to anthrax spores, but it often needs the assistance of the public health authorities to trace a source of supply.

LARVA MIGRANS (Creeping Eruption)

Many intestinal parasites produce larvae which can penetrate the skin of man; usually they migrate via the lungs to the trachea and oesophagus and finish up in the gastrointestinal tract where they breed.

Clinical features   Various forms of ankylostoma wander aimlessly in the dermis causing a raised pink serpentine eruption creeping through the skin at a rate of a few centimetres a day. Larvae of strongyloides extend much faster, up to 10 cm/hr.

  These pruritic burrows (Fig. 14.2) are particularly liable to affect holidaymakers on tropical beaches, children in sand-pits and those who run barefoot in the jungle. Larvae may penetrate the perineal skin after scratching a parasite-induced pruritus ani. All these larvae ultimately die but most patients are not prepared to wait and expect immediate, effective therapy.

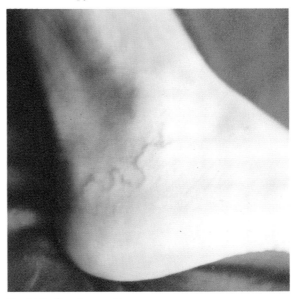

Fig. 14.2   Creeping eruption.

Management   Freezing the skin with carbon dioxide snow, ethyl chloride spray or liquid nitrogen for 2–3 cm around the advancing lesion usually stops the migration. The day after a lesion has been frozen a new one may be seen to branch away from the original burrow. This needs further treatment.

  Patients with many lesions respond well to oral thiabendazole in weekly doses of about 50 mg/kg body weight. This drug has such unpleasant side-effects that it is unkind and unnecessary to use it for solitary lesions. Good results have also been obtained from a 20% suspension of thiabendazole in propylene glycol applied under occlusion daily for a week or so.

LEISHMANIASIS

Clinical features   *Oriental sores:* primary cutaneous leishmaniasis most often develops on exposed skin at the site of a sandfly bite; a red, itchy patch grows slowly, crusts and after 2 or 3 months starts to ulcerate. The lesion is up to several centimetres in diameter and heals within a year, often leaving an unsightly scar. It is common around the Mediterranean, in the Middle East and Pakistan, where it is caused by *Leishmania major* (*L. tropica*)—the desert rat is usually the intermediate host.

Lupoid leishmaniasis (Leishmania recidivans) not all cases of oriental sore resolve completely; sometimes, a tuberculoid granuloma develops in the scar mimicking lupus vulgaris and extending steadily over the face (Fig. 14.3). It is comparable to tuberculoid leprosy in that it shows a high but incomplete host resistance.

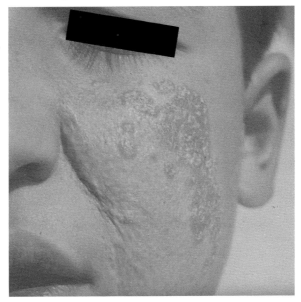

Fig. 14.3   Lupoid leishmaniasis.

Anergic leishmaniasis: in some parts of Africa and South America there are occasional patients whose resistance to the leishmania seems to be non-existent. Many nodules extend across the skin in a condition clinically indistinguishable from lepromatous leprosy. Leishmania are present in considerable numbers in every lesion.

Muco-cutaneous leishmaniasis: seen in equatorial South America and some parts of Central Africa, this is usually caused by *L. brasiliensis.* Its inoculation into the skin produces a nodule clinically similar to the oriental sore. After a varying time the parasite spreads to muco-cutaneous junctions, possibly destroying the larynx, nasal septum, vulva or anus. Most commonly the lips and nose are massively eroded (Fig. 14.4).

Post kala-azar dermal leishmaniasis: L. donovani causes systemic leishmaniasis in which high fever and severe anaemia are combined with gross enlargement of the liver and spleen. The skin darkens and untreated patients die of wasting and intercurrent infection. Some who survive the initial onslaught produce several skin abnormalities in which many nodules erupt, particularly around the mouth and on the chin. These lesions are probably a reservoir of infection from which biting sandflies spread the disease.

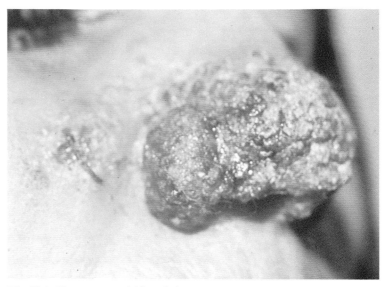

Fig. 14.4 Muco-cutaneous leishmaniasis.

Many other forms of leishmania are known to affect the skin; Ethiopia, Guyana, Mexico, Panama, Peru and other countries have all been found to harbour organisms with delicate biochemical differences. The lesions look like slowly-extending, destructive oriental sores.

Management

All forms of cutaneous leishmaniasis, even the self-limiting oriental sore, should be treated in an attempt to limit mutilation. A search for leishmania should always be made when slowly-extending or ulcerating nodules appear in the persons living in, or who have visited, endemic areas.

Most respond reasonably well to sodium stibogluconate given as 600 mg intravenously or intramuscularly for 2 weeks. Kala-azar needs 4–6 weeks treatment and has to be supplemented with a good diet and treatment for the severe anaemia.

Lupoid leishmaniasis and muco-cutaneous disease may respond slowly to a single course of treatment and repeated courses of sodium stibogluconate at 3-monthly intervals should be given for up to a year.

For anergic leishmaniasis and others not helped by sodium stibogluconate, the unpleasantly toxic drug pentamidine isethionate may be needed. Such patients must be monitored carefully: 3–4 mg pentamidine/kilo bodyweight must be given every 4 or 5 days until well after the clearance of the disease. This drug changes glucose metabolism. Blood sugar estimations (or, preferably, glucose tolerance tests) should be made as often as possible—at least once a week. Careful observation must be maintained for other adverse effects.

A safer but probably less effective substitute for sodium stibogluconate is a 4-week course of rifampicin 1.2 g daily either alone or with 300 mg of isonicotinic acid hydrazide.

Small oriental sores have been treated by surgical excision.

Cryotherapy may be used with a single freeze-thaw cycle, applying the probe until the ice ball has spread a few millimetres outside the lesion for 30 seconds. Lupoid leishmaniasis sometimes responds well to carbon dioxide slush (made by mixing carbon dioxide snow with a small amount of acetone) or liquid nitrogen over the whole area.

If all else fails, intravenous or intramuscular amphotericin B can be tried, long-term.

LEPROSY

Uncomplicated leprosy

Clinical features   Patients develop different clinical presentations according to their personal immunity. Those with high but incomplete resistance produce a few dry scaly anaesthetic patches of tuberculoid leprosy. Those with no resistance develop lepromatous disease; they have many red nodules (nodular lepromatous leprosy) or diffuse lepromatosis—a general skin thickening which may be recognized only when madarosis (loss of eyebrows) draws attention to the skin. Between these two extremes is borderline leprosy with an intermediate number of lesions, some of which are annular. Their number increases in inverse proportion to the resistance (higher resistance, fewer patches).

Hard nodular lesions appear on the peripheral nerves (ulnar, lateral popliteal, great auricular) early and asymmetrically in tuberculoid disease. Lepromatous patients develop anaesthesia of the 'stocking-and-glove' type in the later stages. The severe systemic manifestations of the disease which, if untreated, may lead to mutilation and even death will not be considered here.

Diagnosis depends on the recognition of anaesthesia, the detection of *Mycobacterium leprae* in the skin, or the histopathology of the granulomatous lesions.

Management   Dapsone (di-amino-di-phenyl-sulphone) remains the drug of choice. Patients can be given 100 mg daily with little fear of methaemoglobinaemia or major haemolysis.

Unfortunately, in increasing numbers of patients the *Mycobacterium leprae* are resistant to dapsone. This tragedy may be detected over several years by rising numbers of shiny nodules despite treatment. Earlier diagnosis of dapsone resistance is made from skin smears taken at 6-weekly intervals to monitor changes in the Morphologic Index (the percentage of solidly staining, viable organisms).

Pauci-bacterial patients with tuberculoid disease may still be treated with dapsone alone but all others should receive a combination of drugs in the following regime:
1. Dapsone 100 mg daily indefinitely *plus*
2. A single dose of rifampicin 1500 mg weekly for 4–6 weeks *plus*
3. Clofazimine 100 mg twice daily for 2 months and then daily for 4 more months.

Ethionamide (375 mg daily for 3 months) may also be prescribed but it has many side-effects and it is usually not necessary. In parts of Europe a combination tablet containing isoniazid, prothionamide and dapsone can be obtained.

Tuberculoid patients should continue treatment for 5 years after the complete disappearance of all visible skin lesions—established anaesthesia is unlikely to clear completely. Lepromatous patients should be treated for life; most do not become smear negative for 7–10 years after starting effective therapy but it is most unwise to stop at this time. A few viable 'persisters' sometimes remain, waiting for the opportunity to regain ascendancy over the patient. Also, patients whose lack of resistance has let them develop lepromatous disease may, untreated, become re-infected. Medication for the first 10–12 years is therefore therapeutic—it should be continued as a prophylactic indefinitely.

Patients with sulphone resistance must have rifampicin 600 mg daily for a month plus clofazimine 100 mg daily for life; ethionamide may be added.

Leprosy reactions

Clinical features In lepromatous leprosy, sudden lessening of resistance may cause the lesions to become raised, red and painful. Similar changes in an intra-neural lesion may cause acute wrist-drop, foot-drop, facial palsy or other acute nerve paralysis. This is called the 'reversal reaction' and usually occurs a few weeks after treatment starts.

A similar sudden reaction in pre-existing lesions may occur before antileprosy treatment in which case it may well be why the patient has sought treatment. This is associated with the loss of what small amount of immunity was present and is known as 'downgrading'. In both cases treatment is imperative to prevent permanent nerve palsies.

Management 40–60 mg of prednisolone or its equivalent is given daily for up to two weeks, followed by a slow reduction. Antileprosy therapy must be continued and suitable orthopaedic measures (e.g. cock-up splints) should be taken to help rest damaged peripheral nerves.

Erythema nodosum leprosum

Clinical features When the organisms are killed and slowly disintegrating (a process which takes many years), patients with a high bacterial load may respond with a vasculitis presumed to be a humoral reaction to the release of bacterial toxins. High fever and waves of painful red nodules affecting any part of the skin, including the face (a differentiating point from ordinary erythema nodosum) may persist for many years.

Management Some mild cases are treated with oral chloroquine twice daily, and if it is available, a tri-valent antimonial. Most need long hospitalization.

Erythema nodosum leprosum will not resolve naturally until the bacterial index has become negative, i.e. there are no more organisms. In the past it was treated with long-term steroids and intermittent ACTH.

The recognition that thalidomide has dramatic success in suppressing this reaction has made it the drug of choice for all cases. It should be given 100 mg 2−4 times a day for as long as necessary and suitable precautions should be taken at the same time to prevent patients from becoming parents. Rifampicin may counteract the effect of the contraceptive pill.

1−2 mg of colchicine daily may have a dramatic effect on erythema nodosum leprosum.

Late complications

Nerve lesions of tuberculoid leprosy may cause paralysis and wasting of groups of muscles (Fig. 14.5). When it is quite sure that the disease has been inactivated, orthopedic surgeons can sometimes transpose tendons and return some movement to a previously paralysed hand or foot. Details of such operations are in leprosy textbooks.

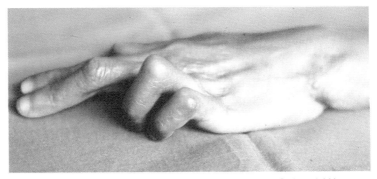

Fig. 14.5 Paralysis and wasting of muscles due to nerve lesions of tuberculoid leprosy.

Ulcers of the feet: leprosy patients must be trained to examine their anaesthetic feet carefully every day for casual unnoticed trauma, ignorance of which may ultimately cause plantar ulcers where sinuses lead down to necrotic fragments of secondarily infected bone. If these ulcers are ignored, persistent infection results in chronic lymphangitis and finally lymphostasis verrucosa cutis or 'mossy foot'. Infection is best prevented by antibiotics and curettage of the ulcers and sinuses to remove necrotic bone. The foot must be encased in plaster and the patient kept in bed until it has healed. after which special footwear should be provided in which Plastozote or microcellular rubber soles ensure that pressure is not on the scar but is evenly distributed across the sole of the foot.

SOME DEEP MYCOSES

These are not to be confused with those dermatophytes and yeasts which live on or in keratin, causing tinea, candidosis, pityriasis versicolour etc. Other fungi or near-fungi inoculated into the dermis by contaminated puncture woulds can set up chronic inflammation.

Chromomycosis

Clinical features This condition extends usually from the dorsum of the foot locally in a warty papular plaque, sometimes clearing in the centre. The lesions may ulcerate. Histologically, there is a tuberculoid granuloma with golden-brown septate spores of Phialophora or Cladosporium.

Management In vitro, these organisms are sensitive to amphotericin B: systemic administration of the drug rarely helps but success may follow intra-lesional injections, weekly, of 2–3 ml of a solution of 50 mg in 20 ml of 5% glucose.

Simpler, and often more effective, is local excision or curettage of small lesions followed by cautery of the base; in the weeks before and after the operation the patient should take a saturated solution of potassium iodide orally in increasing doses (3 drops three times a day increasing slowly to 4 ml three times a day).

Several months' treatment with oral ketoconazole 400 mg daily or 5-fluorocytosine injection every 6 hours may be useful.

Topical heat is very useful; Japanese doctors have recommended local application of a benzene pocket warmer or an electric bed-heater to the lesion for several hours a day.

Sporotrichosis

Clinical features The natural habitat of *Sporotrichum schenckii* is rotting timber and vegetation and it penetrates the skin of the foot on an infected splinter. After a long incubation, crusted erythematous papules develop, to be followed by smaller satellite lesions (Fig. 14.6). The nodules ascend the limb along superficial lymphatics and ulcerated nodules eventually appear over regional lymph nodes.

Management Excision is seldom successful. A saturated solution of potassium iodide may be given orally in increasing doses (3 drops three times a day increasing slowly to 4 ml three times a day, continuing for a month after clinical cure). Local heat is helpful but only before the disease has started to extend.

More expensive and, perhaps, more successful are systemic amphotericin B or ketoconazole given daily for 3–6 months.

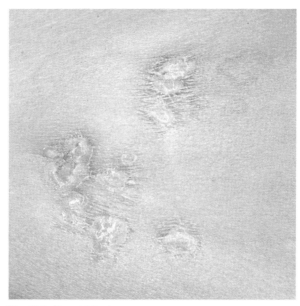

Fig. 14.6 Sporotrichosis.

Madura foot

Clinical features Usually following a penetrating injury a painless nodule appears on the foot which breaks down and becomes surrounded by a mass of nodules and draining sinuses (Fig. 14.7) from an almost completely destroyed inner foot, in which bone absorption produces a completely disabling deformity. Many organisms have been recovered from these lesions—true fungi (madurellae, cephalosporia, phialophora etc) and some

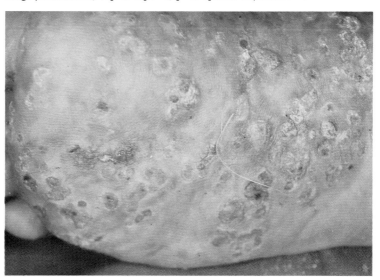

Fig. 14.7 Madura foot.

actinomycetes (*Nocardia braziliensis, Streptomyces madurai*). They tend to produce different coloured granules in the purulent discharge.

Management

Nocardia and Streptomyces respond well to co-trimoxazole tablets twice daily for several months, supplemented if necessary by dapsone 100 mg daily, intramuscular streptomycin or even by systemic penicillin.

These are useless against the fungal forms of madura foot, which may respond to amphotericin B, ketoconazole or 5-fluorocytosine. Many cases resist all medication and the foot has to be amputated. This should be performed as early as possible so that the smallest amount of tissue is removed.

Actinomycosis

Several different actinomycetes affect the skin; one of the more common is *A. israelii*, an anaerobic organism which may live saprophytically in the tonsillar crypts. It sometimes becomes pathogenic in the jaw (by invading the cavity after extraction of a carious tooth), the lung, the caecum and appendix.

Clinical features

A thick, brawny infiltration spreads to neighbouring tissues and invades the overlying skin, giving a board-hard, ill-defined infiltrated plaque (Fig. 14.8). This breaks down to discharge sero-purulent material with golden-yellow granules, wrongly called 'ray fungus'. The disease, once

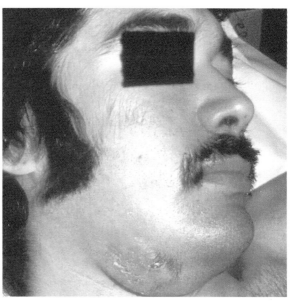

Fig. 14.8 Actinomycosis.

common in Europe, has disappeared from many countries and is diminishing in developing countries.

Management   Penicillin is the drug of choice but at least a million units (600 mg) must be given daily for several months. Excision of sloughing tissue may be indicated. The disease seems sometimes to reactivate (probably from organisms which have been protected by scar tissue) in which case a different antibiotic, preferably tetracycline, should be used in high doses for as long as necessary.

North American Blastomycosis

Clinical features   *Blastomyces dermatitidis* usually affects the skin only secondarily. Spore inhalation causes chronic respiratory infection clinically similar to pulmonary tuberculosis. Following this, often a long time later, infection spreads to the skin. A nodule enlarges, discharges pus and extends peripherally, with warty lesions and micro-abscesses surrounding an atrophic scar. Subcutaneous tissue, bones, joints or the renal tract become affected. Biopsy shows micro-abscesses mixed with chronic tuberculoid granuloma, in which many Langerhan's giant cells each contain several thick-walled spherical yeast cells.

Management   Amphotericin B is useful if the highest tolerated doses are continued until healing is complete, but it is easier to give ketoconazole by mouth, 400 mg a day for several weeks. If the response is not good, treatment can be supplemented with increasing doses of potassium iodide or the systemic use of stilbamidine.

   Any existing deep infection must be recognized and be shown to respond to treatment.

Paracoccidiodomycosis

Clinical features   *Paracoccidioides braziliensis* causes painful granulomata spreading across the mouth to the tonsil and larynx, with dense, red granulations or 'mulberry' erosions. Later the teeth loosen and fall out, regional lymph nodes are infected, enlarge and break down, forming chronic sinuses. Many untreated patients die of systemic complications.

   It can be confused with other deep fungal infections, e.g. rhinosporidiosis or with mucocutaneous leishmaniasis.

Management   It is best to give co-trimoxazole twice daily long-term. If this is not completely successful, ketoconazole 400 mg daily should be prescribed. Injections of amphotericin B are more trouble and no more effective.

ONCHOCERCIASIS

The World Health Organisation estimates that over 40 000 000 people are affected by onchocerciasis, some 1% of whom have been blinded.

Clinical features   Onchocerciasis is an infection with *Onchocerca volvulus*—a thread-like filarial worm in the dermis. They produce enormous numbers of microfilariae which lodge in the skin or eye but only reach maturity in an intermediate host, a black fly of the Simuliidae family. The adult worms live for many years in man but finally die. If the patient escapes further bites from an infected fly, the disease will burn out.

Starting with a severely pruritic dermatitis, large areas of skin become lichenified. Destruction of elastic tissue leaves lax wrinkled skin, 'hanging skin', which often festoons the groin. There are mottled hypopigmented areas (Fig. 14.9). Ultimately clusters of mature worms are surrounded by a fibrous reaction to form firm dermal nodules called onchocercomata, most commonly on the scalp in the Americas and around the pelvic rim in Africans.

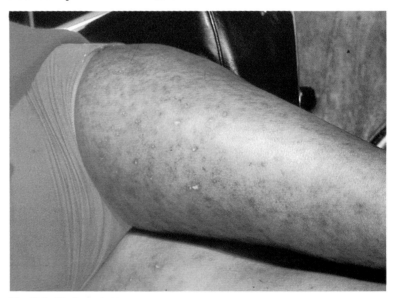

Fig. 14.9 Onchocerciasis.

Management   The diagnosis should be confirmed by taking a skin-snip—a minute 'tent' of skin is raised from the surface by a needle and shaved off without causing any bleeding. The microfilariae can be teased out of the shaving after it is placed in a drop of saline on a microscope slide.

Diethyl carbamazine is the treatment of choice against microfilariae of *O. volvulus*. It must be given with care to minimise the chance of an allergic response aggravating the eye infection. Start slowly with one 50 mg tablet on the first day, two on the second and three on the third. Increase to 100 mg three times a day on the fourth day and then give 250 mg three times a day for a further 10 days. Mydriatics and corticosteroid eye drops should always be available to handle ocular complications.

Suramin may be effective against the adult worms but is useless against microfilariae and is not recommended.

Patients with a limited number of onchocercomata may have them removed surgically. Mass 'nodulectomy' in some areas has been followed by a reduction in new cases.

Outside the riverside areas inhabited by the intermediate hosts, re-infection need not be feared but in endemic regions further courses of treatment may be needed.

SOME TROPICAL ULCERS

The name 'tropical ulcer' is used randomly for any breach of the skin surface which takes a long time to heal. Many different organisms have been found in these ulcers, most of which are surprisingly painless.

Tropical phagedenic ulcers

Clinical features
These painful ulcers spread widely and deeply, producing a foul-smelling discharge. Left untreated they persist for many months or even years and squamous epithelioma may develop. They often contain fusiform bacilli together with the *Treponema vincenti*. There is disagreement as to whether these cause the ulcer or are simply secondary invaders of a devitalized skin but in either case the ulcer will not heal until they have gone. Metronidazole in doses of up to 400 mg three times a day has largely replaced the previous use of systemic penicillin which, in any case, was not invariably useful. Ulcers less than 5 cm in diameter usually heal well. Epithelialization of larger lesions may be encouraged by pinch grafts after infection has subsidised.

Corynebacterial ulcers

Several different corynebacteria have been isolated from ulcers:

Diphtheritic ulcers. These were diagnosed by the presence on the ulcer floor of a membrane which could only be removed with difficulty—some patients had associated diphtheritic paralyses. If diphtheria ever returns in epidemic form it may be expected that these ulcers will re-appear too.

C. pyogenes infection has been found to cause epidemics of ulceration on Thai schoolchildren's legs. The lesions, usually solitary and foul-smelling, differ from tropical phagedemic ulcers by being painless.

Management
Soap and water and local use of Burow's solution (Aluminium Acetate Lotion Aqueous) clear the infection.

Mycobacterium ulcerans infection (Buruli ulcer)

Clinical features
This is the only mycobacterium to produce liquefaction necrosis. The lesions are usually solitary, growing over a major joint. A painless red

nodule forms and quickly breaks down to a large shallow ulcer with
deeply undermined edges (Fig. 14.10).

Management   Surgeons have been known to amputate a limb but this should never be
necessary. There is some disagreement as to which, if any,
antimycobacterial drugs are truly efficacious; clofazimine 100 mg three
times a day and rifampicin 300 mg daily are particularly recommended
but the improvement may be due simply to spontaneous remission.
Isonicotinic acid hydrazide and dapsone are unhelpful but ulcer toilet—
cleaning under the overhanging edge with Eusol or Burow's solution
several times a day—is essential.

The infected joint should be immobilised in plaster of Paris with a
window to permit ulcer toilet. When the granulation tissue on the floor
of the ulcer is healthy and glistening, pinch-grafts can be applied but by
then spontaneous epithelialization is already visible.

Debriding the undermined skin should be discouraged as it usually
reattaches itself to the ulcer floor, reducing the area which needs to be
epithelialized. A cradle with a source of heat over the affected limb for
several hours a day is effective ancillary treatment.

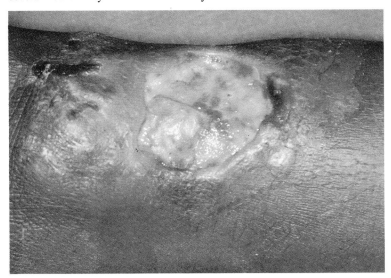

Fig. 14.10 Buruli ulcer.

YAWS

This treponemal disease was once a major public health problem in
many parts of the world but concerted efforts by Unicef and the WHO
were so successful that many people hoped the disease had been
eradicated. Unfortunately, over the past 10 years it has been re-appearing
in many less affluent rural areas in and around the Pacific.

Clinical features   It is caused by *Treponema pertenue*, a spirochaete which is indistinguishable from *T. pallidum* in every way except in the signs and symptoms of the disease it produces. It is contagious among children living in equatorial rain forests whose scanty clothing permits skin-to-skin, non-venereal contact.

The 'mother yaw' is a proliferating, crusting papilloma up to 5–6 cm in diameter which enlarges for a few months then heals with a scar. Blood-borne spread produces red, raspberry-like lesions known as daughter yaws which proliferate, ooze, heal and recur for several years if untreated. Periostitis and swelling of joints in the hands and feet may be linked with painful hyperkeratoses on the soles which make walking difficult. These too finally subside.

After months or even years, late yaws appears with gummata in bones; the tibia shows anterior bowing, bosses develop on the skull and the carpal bones become necrotic. In Africa, nasal septal destruction has been blamed on yaws.

Management   There is no laboratory study to separate *T. pertenue* from *T. pallidum*. Penicillin G should be given (2 mega units—1.2 gm—into each buttock) and all the immediate contacts should be similarly treated. Patients sensitive to penicillin must be given large doses of tetracycline or erythromycin for 3 weeks.

REFERENCES

General
Pettit J H S, Parish L C 1984 Manual of tropical dermatology. Springer Verlag, New York
Anthrax
Dutz W 1981 Anthrax. In: Braude A I (ed) Medical microbiology and infectious diseases, ch 246. Saunders, Philadelphia
Larva migrans
Edelglass J W et al 1982 Cutaneous larva migrans in northern climates. J Am Acad Dermatol 7: 353
Leishmaniasis
Peters W, Evans D A, Lanham S M 1983 Importance of parasite identification in cases of leishmaniasis. J Roy Soc Med 76: 540
Leprosy
Jopling W H 1984 Handbook of leprosy, 3rd edn. Heinemann, London
Chromomycosis
Tagami H et al 1979 Topical heat therapy for cutaneous chromomycosis. Arch Dermatol 115: 740
Mycetoma
Pankajalakshmi V V, Taralakshmi V V 1982 Small grain mycetomas in the tropics. Aust J Dermat 23: 39
Paracoccidioidomycosis
Favre S, Miranda J L, Marques 1974 Clinico-pathological study of oral lesions of South American blastomycosis. Cutis 14: 555
Onchocerciasis
Connor D H 1978 Onchocerciasis, current concepts of pathogenesis. S-E Asian J Trop Med & Pub Hlth 9: 209
Mycobacterium ulcerans
Pettit J H S, Marchette N J, Rees R J W 1966 Mycobacterium ulcerans infection. Brit J Derm 78: 187
Yaws
Browne S G 1982 Yaws. Int J Dermatol 21: 220

W. Frain-Bell

15. The Photodermatoses

It is in relatively recent times that it has become possible to identify clearly those reactions of the skin which are due to exposure to light and to separate them from those resulting from exposure to other factors. This has been due mainly to the development of reliable methods of phototesting, leading to the identification of the responsible wavelengths which, when taken in association with other features, has allowed for a clearer definition of the various photodermatoses. This in turn has made the clinical diagnosis of photosensitivity easier in situations where confirmatory phototesting is not readily available. As a result of this improvement in diagnosis, the treatment and management of cutaneous sensitivity has become more effective.

Thus, effective management is dependent on a correct clinical diagnosis of photosensitivity. Such a diagnosis would be a simple matter if all those so affected complained of an eruption which was confined to the exposed skin, which occurred only during the sunshine months, and which varied in severity with the amount of sunlight exposure. Although this is often what happens, certain of the photodermatoses do vary from this pattern. Also, the changes which occur in the skin are not peculiar to photosensitivity reactions, although some do occur more often in one photodermatosis than in another, as illustrated by the dusky erythema (with or without pigmentation) of drug induced photosensitivity, the prurigo lesion of actinic prurigo, the variable papular erythema of polymorphic light eruption, and the dermatitis or pseudolymphoma changes of the actinic reticuloid syndrome.

Following the identification of the specific photodermatosis, the subsequent management will vary. However, there is the basic requirement for the correct use of topical and systemic photoprotective agents along with access, when necessary, to hospital inpatient care. This allows for nursing in a light protection cubicle which facilitates the suppression of the reactive skin which is often an essential first step in the investigation and subsequent treatment of the photosensitivity response and in the definition of the causal factors.

GENERAL CLINICAL FEATURES

In many of the photodermatoses, much can be learned from the distribution of the eruption. This tends to involve those parts of the skin which are exposed to the maximum amount of sunlight. On the face this is usually prominences such as the nose, cheeks and forehead (Figs. 15.1 and 15.2). On the neck it involves the anterior 'V' with affection particularly over the upper part of the sternoid muscle with a sharp collar cut-off line especially well seen with the shorter hair styles of male subjects. Variations in hair style and stages of constitutional alopecia (Fig. 15.2) provide alterations in distribution which when present are of diagnostic value. In the same way parts of the exposed skin of the arms and legs are more prone to react than others.

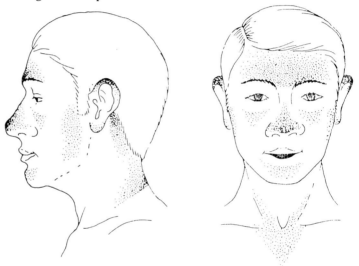

Fig. 15.1 The distribution of cutaneous photosensitivity reactions with the sites most commonly affected indicated by the dots, with relative freedom of the periorbital, submental and retroauricular skin.

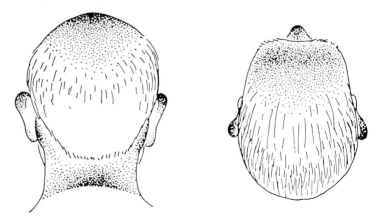

Fig. 15.2 The variable involvement of the scalp in cutaneous photosensitivity in relationship to the type and degree of constitutional thinning. In addition, the distribution of the accompanying reaction on the skin of the ears, neck and nose can be seen.

In certain photodermatoses such as photosensitivity dermatitis and actinic prurigo, the reaction may involve the covered skin also for reasons other than the photosensitivity. It is important to recognise that certain clothes which appear to give adequate protection have spaces in the weave which allow the responsible wavelengths of light to penetrate to underlying skin; this is particularly so when the action spectrum of the photodermatosis involves the longer wavelengths. The cut-off line between a single and a double layer of clothing is a useful physical sign.

It is also important to recognise that the classical photosensitivity distribution, where there is relative freedom of the skin around the eyes, directly behind the ears and under the chin (Fig. 15.3), may be obscured when there are factors additional to that of photosensitivity. As an example, it occurs in photosensitivity dermatitis where a contact allergic component leads to the involvement of one or more of these normally unaffected parts (Fig. 15.4).

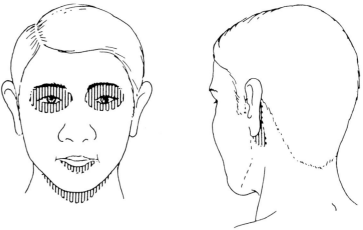

Fig. 15.3 This demonstrates the relative freedom of the periorbital, submental and retroauricular skin which commonly, although not invariably, occurs in cutaneous photosensitivity reactions of the face and neck.

It has been mentioned previously that the skin is limited in the pattern of reactions which it can produce and, therefore, the morphological changes listed in Figure 15.5 are not confined to photosensitivity reactions. Certain combinations of skin changes are, however, more commonly seen in one photodermatosis than in another.

Thus, the clinical diagnosis of a photodermatosis is made by recognising those features which are common to any photosensitivity response and then associating them with those specific to one or other of the photodermatoses.

Polymorphic light eruption

This is the commonest of the idiopathic photodermatoses, although its incidence varies throughout the world being sometimes less frequently seen in those countries with the maximum amount of sunlight. It most

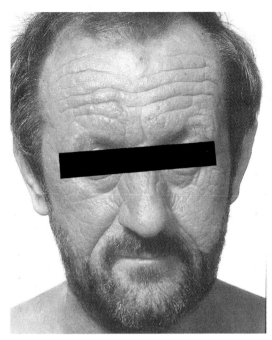

Fig. 15.4 The involvement of the periorbital skin in photosensitivity dermatitis presumably due to the contact allergic component.

commonly affects the female, often—but not invariably—starting in childhood with some suggestion of a familial and atopic background. It presents with a pruritic erythematous reaction of some, although not all, exposed skin sites. The eruption, although often papular, may be any admixture of patches of oedematous erythema, sometimes with an element of urticarial wealing and a tendency in a few adult subjects for the formation of more persistent thickened plaques. In its mild form, polymorphic light eruption is probably more common than the incidence of hospital referral would indicate. It usually lasts for years but in most instances clears up at some stage during adult life. The aetiology and the mechanisms involved in the photosensitivity response are unknown, although the delayed reaction to sunlight, along with the

Erythema
Prurigo
Dermatitis
Scaling/crusting/thickening
Urticaria
Blisters
Scarring
Dyspigmentation
Premalignant changes
Malignancies
Onycholysis
Variations in hair growth and hair colour

Fig. 15.5 The most commonly seen changes occurring in the skin as a result of exposure to light in association or otherwise with abnormal photosensitivity.

lymphocytic infiltration in the skin, suggests a possible involvement of immune mechanisms.

Actinic prurigo

This commonly starts in childhood but usually at an earlier age than in polymorphic light eruption. Although it may continue into adult life, it not infrequently improves during adolescent years. It most commonly affects the female sometimes along with a positive family history for photosensitivity and/or atopy. The main morphological changes are those of a persistent papular/nodular prurigo response in association with episodes of oedematous erythema following exposure of the skin to sunlight (Figs. 15.6 and 15.7). In addition to the maximal involvement of the exposed skin, there is not infrequently a papular prurigo reaction of covered sites. However, the increased reaction of the skin to exposure to sunshine remains an essential diagnostic feature. From time to time some children with actinic prurigo may develop small blisters, particularly on the face, which heal to leave pitted scars.

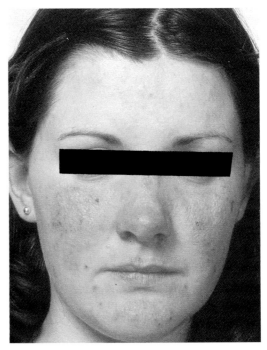

Fig. 15.6

Hydroa vacciniforme

This invariably starts in childhood, is relatively rare and presents as a reaction usually confined to exposed skin in the form of blisters. These can be large and contain clear fluid which subsequently becomes

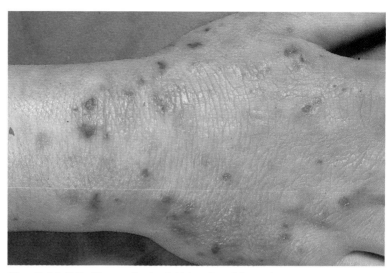

Figs. 15.6 & 15.7   The excoriated and thickened pruriginous skin in actinic prurigo as seen on the face with maximal involvement of the cheeks and distal part of the nose with relative freedom of the skin of the forehead and the sides of the face due to protection from the scalp hair; along with affection of the back of the hand with a sharp cut-off at the wrist.

opalescent. This is followed by an impetiginized crusting phase and ultimately a stage of varicelliform scarring (Fig. 15.8). There is a tendency to slow progressive improvement over the years, often with clearance by late adolescence/early adult life. The mechanisms involved are unknown.

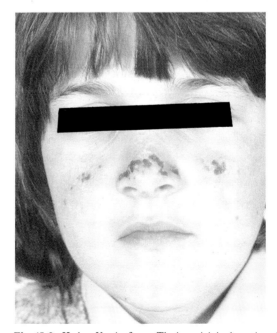

Fig. 15.8   Hydroa Vaccineforme. The impetiginised crusting phase which is resolving to reveal scarring as the crusts separate.

Solar urticaria

This reaction is a relatively rare photodermatosis which presents as short term urticarial wealing of the skin arising soon after exposure to sunshine. The condition tends to last for a variable period of years, the sexes being equally affected, with the majority developing for the first time before the age of 40 years and most doing so in late adolescent and early adult life. As in some subjects with polymorphic light eruption, it may affect maximally parts of the skin normally covered during the winter rather than the exposed skin of the face and backs of hands. Also, a recent solar urticarial response may result in the affected areas becoming less responsive to subsequent exposure. Although the mechanisms involved are not known, it is possible to define specific groups depending on the responsible wavelengths of ultra-violet and visible light in individual subjects (Table 15.1). There is some evidence that immunological mechanisms are involved in those subjects where the action spectrum is confined either to the shorter UVB or to the visible wavebands.

Table 15.1 The identification of different types of solar urticaria based on the wavelengths involved in the urticarial reaction

Type I	Predominantly UVB (290–320 nm)
Type II	Predominantly UVC (320–400 nm)
Type III	Visible light (400–700 nm) or part thereof
Type IV	Wide spectrum (290–700 nm)

Photoaggravated dermatoses (Table 15.2)

Table 15.2 The photoaggravated dermatoses

Atopic Dermatitis
Photosensitive Psoriasis
Lupus Erythematosus
Lichen Planus
Cutaneous Lymphocytoma
Jessner's Lymphocytic Infiltration
Erythema Multiforme
Acne Vulgaris
Pemphigus and Chronic Benign Familial Pemphigus,
Bullous Pemphigoid; Darrier's Disease and
Transient Acantholytic Dermatoses
Disseminated Superficial Actinic Porokeratosis
Pellagra

These are those conditions which are not primarily an abnormal reaction to light but in some subjects have an element of so-called photosensitivity suspected on clinical grounds. The frequency of such photosensitivity varies, perhaps being most commonly present in lupus erythematosus, in which condition the skin changes not infrequently affect particularly those areas of the skin of the face and ears and elsewhere which are maximally exposed to sunlight. In only approximately one-third of these subjects will the action spectrum for erythema be found to be abnormal on phototesting. In psoriasis, lichen planus and erythema multiforme lesions may also take up a photodistribution. This is probably an isomorphic phenomenon and restricted to a few affected subjects who sunburn easily and therefore is not an indication of true photosensitivity. Occasionally, subjects with atopic dermatitis will describe worsening of the reaction of the exposed skin during the summer rather than the more usual aggravation during winter. This is invariably a non-specific aggravation effect of sunlight. The action spectrum for erythema is usually found to be normal on phototesting. Occasionally, atopic dermatitis can be complicated by the development of photosensitivity dermatitis.

The exception is a form of lichen planus, 'lichen planus subtropicus', which occurs in dark skinned subjects and in those parts of the world with maximum amounts of sunshine. The specific diagnostic feature is the development of bluish-brown, scaly, round or oval macules with well-defined borders which in time produce a raised, pale-coloured margin with a relatively depressed brownish centre (Fig. 15.9).

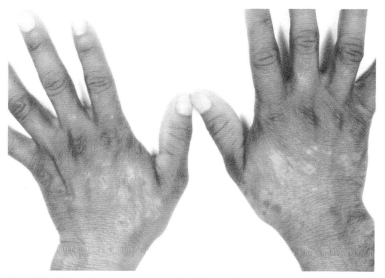

Fig. 15.9   Lichen planus subtropicus. The affection of the skin of the back of the hands with round and oval macules with a well-defined raised pale border and a pigmented centre (patient of Dr Al Fouzan).

Genodermatoses

Of the genodermatoses, those with Bloom's Disease or Rothmund-Thomson syndrome develop changes in the exposed skin which are often poikilodermatous in type and where exposure to sunlight is considered to be partly responsible. The specific effects of ultra-violet radiation are clearly seen in xeroderma pigmentosum, where an inherited enzyme defect leads to impaired repair of UV-damaged DNA, resulting in premature, pre-malignant and malignant degeneration of the exposed skin. In some instances, this may be associated with similar damage to systems other than the skin, as seen in the De Sanctis Cacchione syndrome. A number of complementation groups have now been defined, each with variable characteristics and occurring more commonly in some countries than in others. Although it is a serious condition wherever it occurs, it is more so in those parts of the world where the sunshine exposure factor is high. The variant type of xeroderma pigmentosum is a milder form in which the impairment of repair is of post-replication type and is compatible with a normal duration of life. Thus, it is different from the other complementation groups where the defect is at the stage of excision repair. The clinical presentation is freckling and dryness of the skin developing at any time from adolescence to adult life. There is subsequent premature development in later years of the changes associated with ageing of the skin such as dryness, dyschromia and the premature appearance of solar keratosis, keratoacanthomata and basal cell epitheliomata. This occurs to a lesser extent than in classical xeroderma pigmentosum although some examples do go on to develop squamous cell carcinoma.

The porphyrias

In the porphyrias, cutaneous photosensitivity occurs only if adequate amounts of formed porphyrins collect in the skin where they can absorb wavelengths of long ultra-violet and visible light, leading to the phototoxic-induced skin changes. These will depend on the type of porphyria but in the classical hepatic form (porphyria cutanea tarda), they are usually a combination of blisters and fragility of the skin in association with the formation of milia, dyschromia and increased hair growth. Similar lesions occur in variegate porphyria along with the gastrointestinal and neurological symptoms of the acute intermittent porphyia component.

   The other commonly seen form of porphyria is erythropoietic protoporphyria. This usually starts in childhood and in most instances the symptoms are more severe than any changes in the skin. The affected child experiences extreme discomfort of the exposed skin or, if a young baby, it may scream on being put out in the sunshine. These children, as they grow older, develop ways of lessening this discomfort by, for example, putting their hands under running cold water and if such a history is obtained the diagnosis invariably turns out to be that of erythropoietic protoporphyria. In time, thin linear scars usually develop, best seen on the cheeks and around the mouth. In addition, there is often thickening of the skin over the knuckles and in some instances petechiae may develop, particularly over the backs of the hands. More marked changes occur in those parts of the world where the exposure to sunlight is greater and a marked thickening of the skin can develop. Subjects with this form of porphyria are liable to gallstone formation and hepatic damage.

   In congenital porphyria, which is extremely rare, the photosensitivity reaction eventually leads to tissue destruction. A milder form of congenital porphyria is now recognised where the cutaneous photosensitivity is relatively slight, causing mainly skin fragility and hypertrichosis. Also rare is hereditary coproporphyria in which the presentation is similar to that in variegate porphyria except that abnormal skin changes less often occur, although when they do so they are sometimes severe.

Photosensitivity dermatitis and actinic reticuloid syndrome
(Figs. 15.10, 15.11 and 15.12)

In Britain, this reaction is the most common form of cutaneous photosensitivity to affect males and this may also be the case in some other parts of the world. It most commonly affects middle-aged and elderly males and frequently there is a preceding history of a long-term chronic dermatitis, often of contact type, in which specific allergens may have been demonstrated by skin patch testing. After a variable period of time, usually years, there develops a specific involvement of the photocontact sites. However, in approximately one-third of those affected with photosensitivity dermatitis the mode of onset is that of a photocontact reaction from the start. Where this occurs, the term photocontact dermatitis is often used.

The natural history in both instances is a progression towards a perennial eruption maximally affecting the exposed skin but which may also involve covered skin. This reaction of the exposed skin will usually be found to be worse during the summer. The morphological and histological changes are those of a dermatitis. In a few cases the reactivity of the skin is such that the morphological and histological features, instead of being those of a dermatitis, become instead a pseudo-lymphoma response. This consists of lymphoma-like nodules and plaques, often separated by areas of normal skin and with histological changes in which the cellular response is more pleomorphic than in the dermatitis phase. Also the reaction usually spreads much deeper into the dermis. The involved cells are atypical and may invade the epidermis although they do not form the classical Pautrier microabcesses seen in mycosis fungoides. The two phases of photosensitivity dermatitis and actinic reticuloid syndrome appear to be extremes of a single syndrome and are interchangeable. It is, however, not clear why a pseudo-lymphoma reaction should develop in one individual rather than another when the insults to the skin of both immunological and non-immunological (phototoxic) type appear to be similar. The photosensitivity involves a broad spectrum of wavelengths usually throughout the whole ultra-violet (both UVB and UVA) and not infrequently also into the visible light beyond 400 nm. There is an increased incidence of contact allergy to multiple allergens and, in particular, to the Compositae group of plants and allied compounds and to certain fragrance materials and, possibly, also to other common contact allergens. A number of these contact allergens are capable of producing phototoxic reactions adding to potential sources of skin insult.

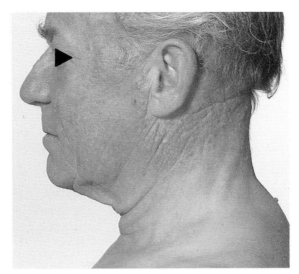

Fig. 15.10

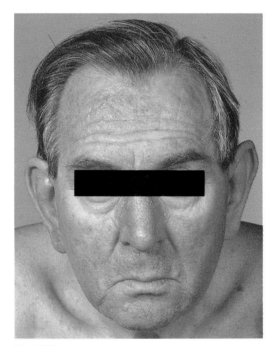

Fig. 15.11

Figs. 15.10, 15.11 & 15.12
Photosensitivity dermatitis and actinic reticuloid syndrome. Some of the morphological
and distribution features of this syndrome, indicating particular involvement of the skin of
the sides of the face, the pinna, the back of the neck and the area over the upper part of the
sterno mastoid muscle (Fig. 15.11) and the pseudo lymphoma changes of the actinic
reticuloid phase (Fig. 15.12).

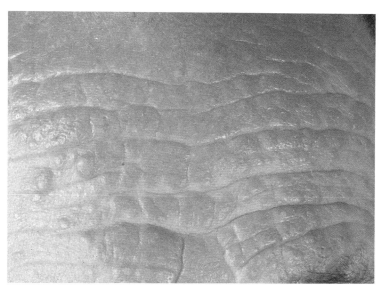

Fig. 15.12

Drug-induced photosensitivity

The incidence of drug-induced photosensitivity is not known. It may be that it is in fact uncommon or, alternatively, that such reactions when they occur are short-lived and may so closely simulate a sunburn erythema that they fail to be recognised as abnormal by the subject and his physician. Such a reaction is, in most instances, of phototoxic type and usually presents as a dusky erythema along with a variable amount of oedema, with or without the subsequent development of pigmentation. In some instances, however, pigmentation may gradually develop without obvious preceding or accompanying erythema. Sometimes the reaction, as with drug-induced photosensitivity from nalidixic acid and frusemide, will be that of variable-sized blisters arising on an otherwise normal skin, or from skin where any background reaction is minimal. This blister formation may be associated with fragility of the skin similar to that seen in porphyria. With certain drugs the initial skin discomfort following exposure to sunlight may be of such severity that further exposure is avoided and thus an eruption does not develop. This was particularly well seen with benoxaprofen photosensitivity.

In most instances, however, drug-induced photosensitivity is usually short-lived and related to the continuing administration of the drug and of exposure to adequate amounts of sunlight. There are some subjects however who, despite discontinuation of the drug, continue to react abnormally to light for longer periods than is usual. This observation is mainly anecdotal without supporting evidence from phototesting. However, chronic photosensitivity of the persistent light reaction type, as occurs in photosensitivity dermatitis, does not appear to usually result from the ingestion of such photoactive substances.

MANAGEMENT

The techniques most commonly used in the investigation of patients with suspected cutaneous photosensitivity are phototesting and skin patch and photopatch testing. In addition, there are the routine biochemical, haematological and immunological laboratory studies; the assessment of the repair of UV-damaged DNA and of the phototoxic potential of a certain substance, with basic light microscopic histological assessment and in certain circumstances ultramicroscopical studies. For the practising clinician, the important techniques are those of phototesting, skin patch and photopatch testing.

Phototesting

Phototesting is the exposure of the skin to measured amounts of irradiation with selected wavebands of the sunshine spectrum (Fig. 15.13) and the the recording of the response and the comparison of this response with that which occurs in the skin of normal non-photosensitive subjects. As a first step, all that is required is to provide irradiation with the whole spectrum from 290–700 nm minus the infra-

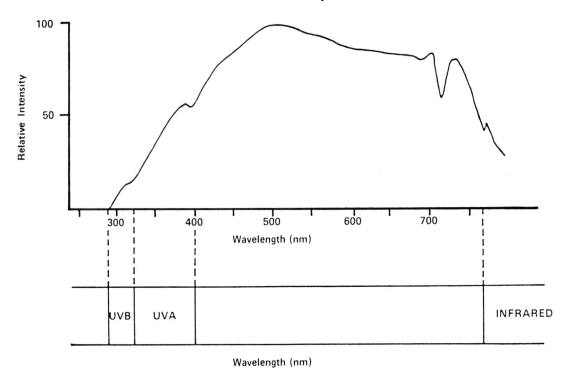

Fig. 15.13   Solar spectrum. The relative intensity of sunshine in relationship to the various wavebands, i.e. UVB (290–320 nm), UVA (320–400 nm) and visible light (>400 nm).

red component (removed by a filter) and a second waveband from which the UVB component (i.e. wavelengths < 320 nm) has been removed by inserting a simple glass filter between the irradiation source and the subject's skin. This screening technique is often sufficient but most subjects with continuing cutaneous photosensitivity will warrant more detailed action spectrum studies whereby the minimal response dose is defined for a range of narrower wavebands throughout the sunshine spectrum. By this technique the clinical diagnosis of cutaneous photosensitivity is confirmed and also the definition of the action spectrum may help to identify a specific photodermatosis and in certain circumstances direct attention towards specific aetiological factors. There are a number of texts, such as that by Johnson and MacKenzie, which deal in more detail with the appropriate irradiation equipment and its use.

Photopatch testing

Although the technique of patch testing is an established and invaluable aid to the assessment of the relevance of contact allergic factors in subjects with dermatitis, it is sometimes difficult to be certain in every instance of the significance of a positive reaction. It is not surprising therefore that, when the skin is exposed to a dose of irradiation of

PHOTOPATCH TEST — CLOSED

Day 1
(a) Determine minimal erythema dose (MED)
(b) Apply patch tests

	non-irradiated control	irradiated
vehicle	○	○
Test Material 1/10	○	○
1/100	○	○
1/1000	○	○

Day 2
(a) Remove patch tests
(b) Irradiate one column. Look for immediate reactions

Day 3 24 hour reading

Day 4 48 hour reading

Day 5 72 hour reading

Fig. 15.14 The photopatch test. The various stages in the conventional photopatch test. The test material concentration will vary.

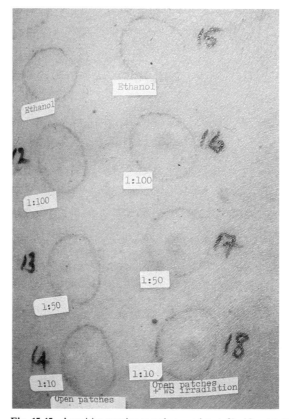

Fig. 15.15 A positive reaction to a photopatch test. Site Nos. 16, 17 and 18 contain increasing amounts of the suspect substance, along with exposure to whole spectrum solar simulator irradiation. This has resulted in a reaction of increasing severity as the amount of the substance is increased from 1:1000 to 1:10, in comparison with no reaction at site Nos. 12, 13 and 14, to which the substance has been applied without subsequent irradiation

variable wavelengths in addition to the chemical substance, the resultant photopatch test reaction may be more difficult to interpret (Figs. 15.14 and 15.15). However, provided certain guidelines are followed, it is a useful test particularly in the assessment of the phototoxic capability of certain substances. It probably tells the clinician more about the photoactive capability of the substance than about the subject's cutaneous photosensitivity.

Management

General measures

Several systemically-administered photoprotective agents are available. Some are effective in certain situations such as in the treatment of the porphyrias. However, the results of treatment in the photodermatoses depend mainly on the measures taken to suppress the reaction and then to maintain the improvement obtained by the regular use of appropriate topical photoprotective agents.

The use of topical corticosteroid preparations by a regimen whereby the strength and frequency of application is reduced in parallel with clinical improvement is more effective in some photodermatoses than in others, particularly so in photosensitivity dermatitis. However, it will be effective only if further exposure to light is avoided or at least minimized. In the more severe forms of photosensitivity, initial nursing behind photoprotective blinds will be needed. These blinds, which can be rolled back to the ceiling attachment when not in use, are made from materials which screen off most of the relevant wavelength of UV and visible light, yet allow the patient to see and be seen easily through the material. The suppression of the reaction will then allow for investigation of the photosensitivity (by means of phototesting and patch and photopatch testing) to proceed without the production of an unwanted excited skin response which invariably occurs if these investigations are started prematurely, i.e. in the presence of a reactive skin. The suppression of the reaction also reduces the possibility of the subject's skin being intolerant to the topical photoprotective agent which at that stage should preferably be of the total block, titanium dioxide type. This preparation can be changed to a more specific and more cosmetically acceptable one once the action spectrum has been defined.

Patients do not always appreciate the amount of unwanted radiation which can reach the skin either by reflection, from sky-shine or through water or window glass and thin clothing; also, that UV exposure is maximum around the middle of the day (11.00 hrs–15.00 hrs) when the sun is at its highest and at the shortest distance from the earth. Despite a reduction in the UVB sunburning component during the second half of the day, there is still a large amount of the longer wavelength UVA around and this may well accentuate the UVB induced-response and, of course, these longer wavelengths are important in many of the photodermatoses. Advice with regard to these factors is an important support to the more specific therapy.

The appearance of the eruption on parts of the skin apparently covered by clothing can be due to light penetration of certain fabrics. Such an effect was noted by the author in 40% of polymorphic light eruption subjects. A reaction of the skin may occur even under thick clothing since the thickness is less important than the structure of the weave, i.e. the closeness of the fibre. The fact that certain parts of the skin are at risk despite being covered by clothing is of importance not only in the clinical diagnosis of the photosensitivity but also in the guidance given with regard to photoprotection. This is true for the photosensitive subject as well as for those who have been temporarily photosensitized by PUVA and other forms of phototherapy.

Topical photoprotective agents

In the treatment of cutaneous photosensitivity, the selection and use of topical photoprotective agents is particularly important. These require to be chosen for their ability to protect against the wavelengths of UV and/or visible light known to be responsible for the eruption as defined by phototesting. They may contain more than one substance so as to be

Table 15.3 Photoprotective agents

Agent	Protect against
Para-aminobenzoic acid (PABA) and esters	UVB
Cinnamates	UVB
Benzophenones	UVB and UVA
Salicylates	UVB
Anthranilates	UVB and UVA
Titanium dioxide and zinc oxide	UVB/UVA/Visible

able to provide a broad spectrum of protection. Table 15.3 illustrates some of the light screening substances currently available and the wavelength cover they provide. In addition to the necessity for protection against a variable-sized waveband, some individuals will require more protection than others on account of a greater degree of photosensitivity. The relative degree of protection provided by different preparations against the sunburning component of sunlight is defined on the basis of protective factors (PF) or sun protective factors (SPF): for example, PF5 will protect against exposure to approximately 5 minimal erythema doses (MEDs) for a specific waveband. Using a range of protective factors it is possible to vary the degree of protection within a group of individuals who may have the same type of photodermatosis but differ in the severity of the UV sensitivity.

The substances listed in Table 15.3 have been selected for their ability to absorb certain wavelengths as demonstrated by a spectrophotometric definition of their absorption spectrum (Fig. 15.16). This provides only an indication as to how effective a preparation is likely to be once it has been applied to the skin. It is the behaviour of the substance and its vehicle on, and in, the skin which is of importance in determining the protective effect. Much depends on the absorption, whether a depot is

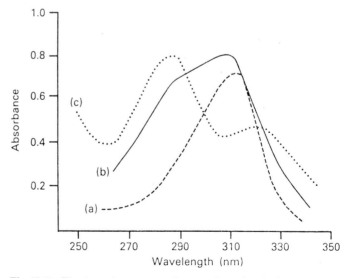

Fig. 15.16 The absorption spectrum of commonly-used, topically applied, photoprotective substances such as para-aminobenzoic acid ester (a), a cinnamate (b) and a benzophenone (c).

created or not and whether the action is affected by washing, sweating, friction and heat.

The clinician should select a small number of photoprotective agents. All that is required is one which will protect against UVB, one which will protect against UVB and UVA, and one which has a block action against a broad spectrum of UV and visible light. It is preferable that they should be free from fragrances and other materials which might produce a phototoxic reaction and from those which are potentially allergenic.

For protection against UV wavelengths, the most effective combination is probably a para-aminobenzoic acid (PABA) ester plus a benzophenone. The former protects particularly well against UVB wavelengths and the latter provides protection throughout UV wavelengths and includes part of the longer wavelength UVA. PABA esters have the advantage of producing a depot of the substance in the skin and being more resistant than some to sweating and swimming. A total block is provided by substances such as titanium dioxide and zinc oxide and much can now be done to make these more cosmetically acceptable. The cinnamates are widely used for protection against the shorter UVB wavelengths but need to be combined with a benzophenone or zinc oxide for the wider protection of the whole UV spectrum.

Many chemical substances are capable of producing a contact allergic reaction and those used for light protection are no exception. Some of the PABA esters produce contact allergic reactions more commonly than seems to occur with the cinnamates or with the benzophenones, although some PABA esters such as octyl dimethyl PABA are less allergenic than others. PABA contains a para-amino group and, therefore, the potential for cross-sensitivity is that much greater. Such allergenic materials are therefore best avoided in the treatment of the state of persistent light reaction of the photosensitivity dermatitis and actinic reticuloid type, in view of the relationship between the chronic photosensitivity and contact allergic sensitivity. Under certain circumstances, these photoprotective chemicals can produce phototoxic reactions and this possibility requires consideration when an otherwise appropriate light screening preparation appears to be ineffective.

Systemic photoprotective agents
None of the systemic photoprotective agents has been shown to be effective except for beta-carotene and the antimalarials and these only in certain situations. Beta-carotene is effective in the treatment of erythropoietic protoporphyria although whether this preparation has much to offer in the treatment of any of the other photodermatoses is debatable and the evidence conflicting. It acts probably on the photosensitivity reaction once it is established in the skin rather than by any photoprotective action. In erythropoietic protoporphyria for example, the assumption would be that it minimizes the effect of the phototoxic reaction rather than acting as a built-in photoprotective agent relative to its absorption spectrum. It is usual now to prescribe a beta-carotene/canthaxin mixture which appears to be equally effective in

providing adequate serum levels but the skin discolouration which it produces is cosmetically more acceptable than that resulting from beta-carotene alone.

The antimalarial drugs, quinacrine, chloroquine and hydroxychloroquine, have been widely used in the treatment of cutaneous photosensitivity. Since there is no evidence that they alter significantly the normal sunburn erythema response in the skin, or have a sunscreening action, interest is mainly centred on their involvement in the mechanisms responsible for abnormal cutaneous photosensitivity response. As with other systemic photoprotective drugs, reports of the efficacy of the antimalarials are based mainly on clinical impressions. Although quinacrine produces more cutaneous side-effects than chloroquine and hydroxychloroquine, the latter two have significant disadvantages in that they can produce irreversible retinal damage which appears to be dose-related. It would seem reasonable for this group of drugs to be used only in cutaneous photosensitivity when other measures have failed.

Systemic corticosteroid therapy is rarely required in the treatment of cutaneous photosensitivity. It is best avoided in chronic photosensitivity since those subjects with, for example, photosensitivity dermatitis and actinic reticuloid syndrome, may become dependent on such treatment particularly if more appropriate measures are not applied at the same time. The correct use of a topical corticosteroid regimen where the amount of treatment is reduced in parallel with clinical improvement, is an essential ingredient in the suppression of the active phases of most of the photodermatoses and is particularly effective in photosensitivity dermatitis.

It will be found that these general measures require to be modified with varying emphasis in the treatment of individual photodermatoses.

Specific measures

Polymorphic light eruption

Most individuals who suffer from this form of cutaneous photosensitivity manage to minimize the response to sunlight by the correct use of topical photoprotective agents with graded exposure to sunlight. Gradually the factor of hardening, peculiar to this photodermatoses, takes over as the summer progresses. This is not always the case and certain sufferers from polymorphic light eruption develop more severe reactions as a result of continuous exposure and may require to maintain full topical photo-protection. This should cover the whole ultra-violet waveband, both UVB and UVA, although protection against the UVB component may be all that is required in those who have a relatively mild form, thus allowing for the development of protective UVA induced pigmentation. There is a group of subjects with polymorphic light eruption who will require more active measures and the treatment of choice in this situation would be either UVB phototherapy or psoralen photochemotherapy.

Actinic prurigo

Treatment is similar to that required in polymorphic light eruption except that sufferers from this photodermatoses are often intolerant of topical photoprotective agents because of the continuing prurigo reaction in the skin. It may be necessary for an initial period of inpatient treatment with nursing in a light protection cubicle with topical corticosteroids to allow tolerance to topical photoprotective agents covering the whole UV waveband. These subjects will also require similar topical corticosteroid therapy to the covered site prurigo reaction. In those most severely affected, relatively short periods of inpatient treatment may be required from time to time. Thalidomide is said to be effective, although the past history of this drug has stood in the way of a more widespread assessment of its efficacy.

Hydroa vacciniforme

Individuals with this form of cutaneous photosensitivity require broad spectrum photoprotective agents and some suggest that betacarotene may also be helpful. In both hydroa vacciniforme and actinic prurigo topical photoprotective agents may not be as effective as in polymorphic light eruption. The reason for this is not clear.

Solar urticaria

It is not possible on clinical grounds to determine which form of solar urticaria is likely to be associated with specific parts of the solar spectrum. Topical photoprotective agents should provide a broad spectrum of protection throughout the ultra-violet and visible light and as such require to be of the block type, perhaps containing also absorbing chemicals appropriate to the UVB and UVA component.

Topical photoprotective agents do not seem to be as effective in solar urticaria as they are in some of the other idiopathic photodermatoses such as in polymorphic light eruption. In most instances, if the urticarial condition is troublesome, treatment with psoralen photochemotherapy is indicated. Whether some of the newer antihistamines will prove to be effective in solar urticaria remains to be seen.

The treatment of the photoaggravated dermatoses is the prophylactic use of topical photoprotective agents which maximally protect against the shorter wavelength UVB, particularly if the individual is fair-complexioned and liable to excessive sunburn reactions. In lupus erythematosus, all those affected, particularly with the systemic variety but also whenever possible in those with cutaneous discoid lupus erythematosus lesions, should use appropriate broad spectrum ultra-violet protective preparations during the sunshine months. Winter-time exposure to sunlight, especially with reflection from snow and ice, should not be forgotten.

The genodermatoses

There is little recorded experience of the suspected photosensitivity factor in the various genodermatoses and the action spectrum for any abnormal reaction in these conditions is essentially unknown. Once the diagnosis is suspected, continuous topical photoprotective agents should be used in the hope that skin changes will be minimized. The exception is xeroderma pigmentosum in which it is essential that continuous total protection from sunlight should be started as soon after birth as possible and continued throughout life with the hope that by so doing the malignant degeneration induced by ultra-violet exposure will be lessened.

Photosensitivity dermatitis

The treatment of photosensitivity dermatitis is directed first of all towards suppressing the reaction which may involve both exposed and covered skin. The basic requirement is for a reduction in sunlight exposure and in those most severely affected this requires hospital treatment with nursing in a light protection cubicle. Phototesting and patch testing can then be carried out without increasing the reactivity of the skin (producing the 'angry back' syndrome) and the affected skin will later tolerate topically applied photoprotective agents. The protective function of the blind material removes the requirement of a topical photoprotective agent until the reaction of the skin has been suppressed. This can be achieved quickly by the use of a reducing-strength topical corticosteroid regimen whereby the potency is reduced in parallel with clinical improvement. The patient is then allowed out of the cubicle for progressively increasing periods each day while wearing a block type of topical photoprotective agent containing titanium dioxide. This is usually well tolerated and has the advantage that it does not contain photoactive or allergenic substances. From time to time such a regimen may be required for the individual patient over a period of years. The requirement will depend on the severity of the reaction and the multiplicity of the factors involved in the production of the chronic reactive process in the skin. If such a regimen is followed it will be rarely necessary for drugs such as azothiaprine or systemic corticosteroids to be used.

Drug-induced photosensitivity

In most instances drug therapy can be continued provided exposure to bright sunlight is reduced and that appropriate topical photoprotective agents which protect against the whole ultra-violet waveband are applied regularly.

FURTHER READING

Johnson B E, Mackenzie L A 1982 Techniques used in the study of the photodermatoses. Seminars in Dermatology 1: 217

J. A. Cotterill

16. Psychogenic Dermatoses

Psychiatric problems may present to the dermatologist with either symptoms referrable to the skin, abnormal dermatological physical signs or both. The physician must be constantly alert to the possibility of dermatitis artefacta. Cutaneous delusions involving the hair, face and perineum are quite common in patients in dermatological clinics and much more common than delusions of parasitosis. In patients with artefact dermatitis and delusional states involving the skin, clear psychiatric pathology can sometimes be delineated. The starting point of management in all these situations is diagnosis.

DERMATITIS ARTEFACTA

Clinical features

Clinical pointers to dermatitis artefacta include a female patient, usually younger than 35 years old, with thick case notes, often containing data of other simulated disease. Others include a hollow history in that the patient cannot describe how the lesion or lesions evolved. Indeed, the presence of fully developed lesions is an important diagnostic feature. The lesions are usually bizarre (Fig. 16.1) and are characteristically in readily accessible sites (Fig. 16.2.). A haemorrhagic crust is typical (Fig. 16.3) and the lesions heal rapidly with simple local treatment, including occlusion, as long as the patient has no opportunity to attack the skin again. Isolated blisters on the legs are a common presentation of artefact dermatitis in adolescent girls.

Management

It must be remembered that the patient with artefact dermatitis is trying to deceive physician, friends and family but it is usually impossible to be sure of the level of the patient's psyche at which the deception is occurring. The abnormal physical signs on the skin are best regarded as a plea for help. It is pointless confronting the patient with the fact that the lesions are self-induced. This may only lead to an angry interchange and the patient will walk out, never to be seen again. Some sort of rapport should be developed with the patient then contact, once established,

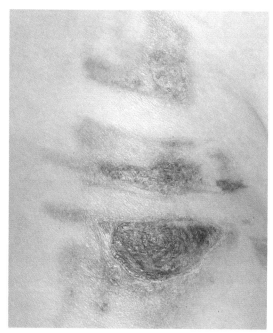

Fig. 16.1 Dermatitis artefacta (typical lesion).

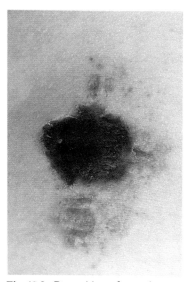

Fig. 16.3 Dermatitis artefacta on leg showing haemorrhagic crust.

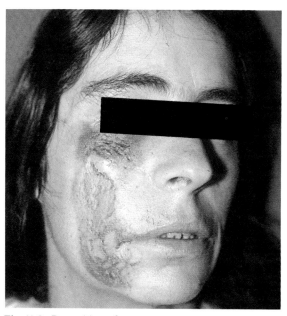

Fig. 16.2 Dermatitis artefacta.

should be maintained. Indeed, the patient should learn that she can attend for consultation without the need to produce the lesions. It is a mistake to discharge the patient as soon as her skin gets back to normal.

Artefact dermatitis in younger girls often responds to manipulation of problems at home. This usually means manipulating mother to the patient's wishes. Whenever possible the background should be fully explored with the parents. From time-to-time there may be other anxieties, such as an unwanted pregnancy, sexual threats of boyfriends, being sent away to school, etc. Often simple reassurance and occlusive bandaging is effective as concern over these, often temporary, upsets recedes.

The older female patient with a long history of artefact dermatitis, often with other forms of simulated disease, has a very poor prognosis. The case notes usually show repeated admissions to hospital, psychiatric units, sometimes alcohol and drug abuse or drug overdoses. Some patients eventually kill themselves.

Psychiatrists may not be particularly helpful in managing patients with dermatitis artefacta. Patients resist going to see a psychiatrist but the dermatologist should not hesitate to involve the psychiatrist if the disturbances appear profound.

ACNE EXCORIÉE

Clinical features   The clinical features of acne excoriée are shown in Figure 16.4. There is usually little difficulty in making the diagnosis. Small acneiform spots are excoriated by the finger nails. Some patients will deny that they have excoriated the lesions which are usually confined to the forehead, face, shoulders, upper back and upper arms. They heal characteristically with

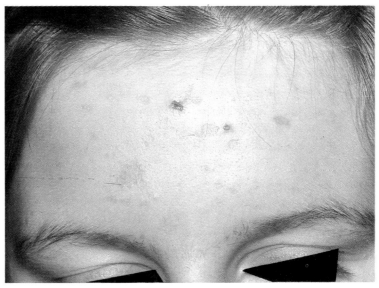

Fig. 16.4   Acne excorieé.

small, white atrophic scars. The clinical spectrum ranges from the anxious teenage female manipulating her acne spots, to habitual skin excoriators.

Management   The management is not easy. It has been claimed that acne excoriée is a protective device to let the patient escape from painful life situations. Psychotherapy to give the patient insight may ultimately produce an anxious, phobic patient. It is therefore probably important that the dermatologist does not cure the patient.

Some patients respond to a small dose of trifluoperazine, such as 1 or 2 mg in the morning. An anxious teenager manipulating frankly acneiform spots can be helped by conventional antibiotic treatment for acne (see Ch. 3).

TRICHOTILLOMANIA OR PATHOLOGICAL HAIR PULLING

Clinical features   Pathological hair pulling is seen more often in boys under 6 years old but is twice as common in girls and women thereafter. It presents from very early childhood to quite late in life. The alopecia produced may be either localized or diffuse (Fig. 16.5) and is engendered by hair twisting, which is commoner in children, or by scissors or a razor, often in the older patient. The fact that the ends of the hairs have been cut can readily be established with a magnifying glass or low-powered microscope. The main differential diagnosis is from alopecia areata in which there are exclamation mark hairs and possibly nail changes (see Ch. 20).

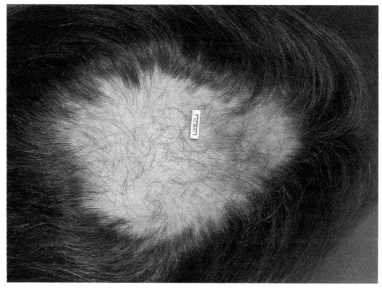

Fig. 16.5   Alopecia produced by trichotillomania.

Management   This is along lines exactly similar to those of the patient with artefact dermatitis. The background to trichotillomania is very simiar to that of artefact dermatitis. The very young child can be given a small bunch of hair to stroke the skin around the head and neck. This is comforting to the child and diverts the fingers from further hair twisting and pulling. In most children recovery is spontaneous.

In older females the prognosis is much poorer. A wig occasionally helps to prevent manipulation of the hair. However, teenage patients often attack their hair in bed at night. Some advocate collodion applied directly to the scalp to try to make this more difficult.

DELUSIONS OF PARASITOSIS

Clinical features This is an unshakable conviction by the patient that he or she is infested by parasites. It is commonest in females after the age of 50. It is unusual to see skin lesions but there may be one or two excoriation marks. The commonest presenting physical signs are the little parcels of debris in plastic bags or matchboxes which the patient thinks contains the parasites! These are usually handed over to the dermatologist. A shared delusion (folie à deux, trois, quatre etc.) is quite common so several members of the same family may become affected. The syndrome is commonly triggered in a rather isolated, obsessional female by frank infestation such as an attack of scabies in one member of the family.

Other pointers to the diagnosis are in the patient's home. On entering the house there is usually a strong smell of antiseptic and a magnifying glass almost always lies on the table. A strong metal comb is used on the scalp to produce little spheres after the hair has been washed. The patient interprets these tiny pieces of epidermis as eggs. The local authority disinfestation team will have visited the house on several occasions; an entomologist from the local university or from the natural history museum and even commercial pest destruction companies may all have been contacted to collude in the delusion. The patient, by the time she is seen, is exhausted from all the washing and cleaning she is doing and other family members are often distraught. The patient can sometimes be actively considering suicide.

Management Management of this delusion requires much tact and skill. It involves both the patient and the other members of the family. The delusion is not uncommon among doctors and its appearance in a medical colleague may pose special difficulties. Delusions of parasitosis can arise in younger patients either from drug addiction or as folie à deux.

It is wise to make sure that there is no underlying organic disease and absolutely vital to exclude a true parasitosis.

Drug therapy with pimozide has revolutionized the management of this condition in truly psychotic patients. This drug, which in most patients has a mildly stimulant effect, is given in the morning in an initial dose of 2 mg daily. It is increased by 2 mg increments weekly until the maximum of 8 or 10 mg is reached. Higher doses produce extrapyramidal symptoms which are not well tolerated. If the patient is not keen on this approach, depot neuroleptics can be used.

Patients with predominantly depressive symptomatology do better on antidepressants using conventional doses of, for example, amitriptyline or dothiepin. Other patients seem to need both pimozide and amitriptyline.

Unfortunately, drug therapy is usually needed for the rest of the patient's life. It is common, however, for compliance to be poor and it is easy to lose touch with the patient.

Dermatologists probably see more patients with this disorder than psychiatrists, for the truly deluded patient takes a suggestion to visit a psychiatrist very badly.

It is most important to be careful what you say to the patient. If pressed whether the parasites are present or not, it is best to say, 'I can't see any today'. It is also polite to agree to examine the debris that the patient almost inevitably brings with him.

DELUSIONS INVOLVING BODY IMAGE

Clinical features   Some patients, mainly female, present to the dermatological clinic with no significant objective skin pathology but with many skin-related symptoms. Complaints are confined to three main body areas.

Dysmorphophobia   Dysmorphophobia is preoccupation with some minor bodily defect which a person thinks is conspicuous to others when, objectively, there is no cause at all for complaint. The most usual facial symptom is burning or excessive redness. Morbid pre-occupation with imagined facial hair is common. It often follows a chance remark by a relative or neighbour. The patient then spends most of her day in front of a magnifying mirror with tweezers, producing folliculitis around the mouth. Centres for electrolysis are familiar with patients who ask for facial hair to be removed when, in reality, there is nothing there. Some patients complain of facial scarring while others become very disturbed about minute telangiectases on their cheeks or nose. Patients with dermatological non-disease sometimes also complain of a burning feeling (orodynia) inside their mouth, often worse at the end of the day and made worse by an acidic food or drink.

Scalp symptomatology   Scalp symptoms consist of complaints of itching and burning, often coupled with anxiety about excessive loss of scalp hair. Females predominate.

Perineal symptomatology   Symptoms referrable to the perineum include severe discomfort, making it very difficult to sit down. Male patients generally older than those with frank facial or scalp symptoms are more represented in this group.

A history of trauma to the back or of spinal or disc disease is common and there may also be a history of local trauma to the skin. In younger men the symptoms may follow imagined or real exposure to potential sexually transmitted disease. Another common complaint in males is of an irritable, red, burning scrotum, the discomfort often spreading to the suprapubic area and to the thighs (see Ch. 12). The patients tend to visit a large number of consultants. One patient is known to have seen at least 27 doctors about his problem, including an orthopaedic surgeon, who divided the lateral cutaneous nerve of the thigh in an attempt to relieve the discomfort. Unfortunately the operation was unsuccessful.

Management   This syndrome is one of the most difficult and time-consuming to manage in dermatology. Patients with dermatological non-disease may have a variety of psychiatric problems, from senile dementia to schizophrenia and depression, but most are moderately or severely depressed. Conventional antidepressants, such as amitriptyline or dothiepin are not often very helpful. The patients often say they are sleeping better and feeling a little happier but that their hair is coming out or that their face is still burning. The response to pimozide is very disappointing but a small group of patients seem to be helped by it. Psychiatrists are no more adept than dermatologists at dealing with the clinical situation.

The major problem is that female patients with facial symptoms either try to commit suicide or manage to do so successfully. Most truly psychotic patients with delusions, for instance, about their nose, should be referred to a psychiatrist, whatever their protestations.

Psychiatric problems presenting to the dermatologist are usually much easier to diagnose than to treat. Pimozide has been a great leap forward in patients with delusions of parasitosis but often all that can be done is to maintain contact with the patient.

FURTHER READING

Cotterill J A 1983 Psychodermatology. Seminars in Dermatology ii(3):
Cotterill J A 1983 Psychiatry and skin disease. In: Rook A J, Maibach H I (eds) Recent Advances in dermatology. Churchill Livingstone, Edinburgh, pp. 189–212
Lyell A 1983 The Michelson Lecture. Delusions of parasitosis. British Journal of Dermatology 108: 485–499
Sneddon IB 1979 The presentation of psychiatric illness to the dermatologist. Acta Dermato-Venerologica 59: suppl. 85, 177–179

R. C. Holmes

17. Pregnancy Dermatoses

INTRODUCTION

Factors which make the management of dermatoses in pregnancy difficult include the confused terminology, concern over the foetal prognosis and the constraints which pregnancy places upon treatment. Of these the confused terminology is the source of most management problems. Recent improvements in classification (Table 17.1) will allow a more confident approach to management. (Particular care must be taken during pregnancy in prescribing any drugs, whether for topical or systemic administration).

Table 17.1 Classification of the dermatoses of pregnancy

Dermatitis	Old terminology	Incidence
Pruritus gravidarum	—	18%
Polymorphic eruption of pregnancy	Toxaemic rash of pregnancy Late onset prurigo of pregnancy Pruritic urticarial papules and plaques of pregnancy Toxic erythema of pregnancy	0.5%
Prurigo of pregnancy	Prurigo gestationis of Besnier Early onset prurigo of pregnancy	0.3%
Pruritic folliculitis of pregnancy		Unknown (probably common)
Pemphigoid gestationis	Herpes gestationis	0.002%
Pustular psoriasis of pregnancy	Impetigo herpetiformis	Unknown (very rare)

CUTANEOUS PHYSIOLOGICAL CHANGES

Pigmentation

An increase in pigmentation is seen in pregnancy, particularly in brunettes. This is especially observable in the areolae, genital skin and the linea alba. A deepening of colour is seen also in skin which is already pigmented. Up to 70% of women develop chloasmal pigmentation in the second half of pregnancy. Symmetrical patches are seen on the forehead, temples and central part of the face. Most cases fade completely after delivery. Increased numbers of pigmented naevi may be noted.

Increased hair loss

This may be seen immediately post-delivery and, in some cases, severe loss may occur 3–4 months later. Complete recovery occurs spontaneously.

Spider naevi

These develop in up to 70% of women between the second and fifth months of pregnancy and can be expected to regress within the 3 months following delivery.

PRURITUS GRAVIDARUM

Clinical features By far the most common skin problem in pregnancy is simple pruritus. It affects approximately one in five women and may be confined to the abdomen or generalized. The skin looks normal apart from excoriations.

Management Management depends on its severity which ranges from mild to intractable with sleep disturbance. In mild cases, calamine cream or lotion usually suffices but they can be supplemented by an oral antihistamine. Antihistamines appear to be free of adverse effects on the foetus, although it is probably safer to prescribe those, such as chlorpheniramine, with which we have the longest clinical experience.

The pathogenesis of pruritus gravidarum is generally attributed to cholestasis and the pruritic effect of bile salts. Cholestyramine may be prescribed for severe intractable cases. This ion-exchange resin binds bile salts in the intestine and limits their entero-hepatic circulation. The degree of cholestasis in pruritus gravidarum varies considerably and only a small minority of patients develop abnormalities in their routine liver function tests. Those with more profound cholestasis must have their pregnancies closely supervised as they have an increased frequency of premature labour, low-birth weight infants and post-partum haemorrhage.

After delivery the pruritus settles rapidly. It may recur in subsequent pregnancies or on taking an oestrogen-containing oral contraceptive. Patients with cholestasis in pregnancy have an increased frequency of gallstones in the long term.

POLYMORPHIC ERUPTION OF PREGNANCY (PEP)

Clinical features   Other names for PEP are 'toxaemic rash of pregnancy' and in the United States, 'pruritic urticarial papules and plaques of pregnancy'. It most commonly begins in the last trimester or immediately post-partum. Realization that its morphology varies considerably as it develops has done much to clarify the classification of pregnancy dermatoses.

At the onset patients develop pruritic erythematous papules usually on the lower abdomen in association with striae (Fig. 17.1). The eruption may extend to resemble a toxic erythema with individual lesions of papules, target lesions and tiny vesicles. As it resolves, the eruption becomes eczematous, with fine crusting and a scaly erythema. Acral papules and vesicles may be seen in about a quarter of the patients. Its varied morphology causes PEP to be frequently misdiagnosed and treated inappropriately. The disorders for which PEP is most commonly mistaken include drug eruptions, erythema multiforme, scabies, eczema and pemphigoid gestationis (herpes gestationis). Features which may be helpful in differentiating PEP and PG are listed in Table 17.2. The precise cause of PEP is unknown but it appears to be an inflammatory response to the formation of striae.

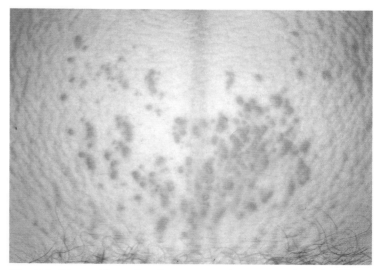

Fig. 17.1 Polymorphic eruption of pregnancy—erythematous papules on the abdomen in association with striae.

Management   Management is directed towards relieving symptoms while awaiting spontaneous resolution. In the average case this can be expected within 6 weeks of onset. The eruption is rarely severe for more than 1 week. Symptoms are usually relieved by a corticosteroid cream and a systemic antihistamine. In the most florid cases, short courses of prednisolone, in a tapering regimen starting at 30 mg daily, will resolve the eruption quickly. It is particularly important to reassure the patient that this is exceedingly common with no adverse effect on the foetus. It does not appear to recur significantly in subsequent pregnancies nor to be associated with other medical disorders.

PRURIGO OF PREGNANCY

Clinical features

This usually begins between 25 and 30 weeks of gestation. It consists of prurigo papules, predominantly on the extensor surfaces of the limbs (Fig. 17.2), termed 'prurigo gestationis of Besnier' and 'early onset prurigo of pregnancy' (Table 17.1). Its aetiology is obscure but it may be the result of pruritus gravidarum in atopic individuals.

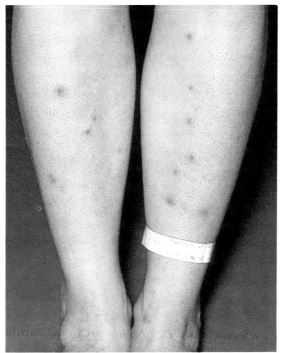

Fig. 17.2 Prurigo of pregnancy—papular lesions on the shins.

Management

Symptomatic control often proves difficult but, fortunately, the itch usually settles promptly after delivery. Prurigo papules may persist for several months post-partum. The foetal prognosis appears normal.

'Papular dermatitis of pregnancy' refers to a syndrome of widespread prurigo lesions, low urinary chorionic gonadotrophin levels and an apparently high fetal loss. Whether this truly represents a distinct disorder or, as seems more likely, simply florid cases of prurigo of pregnancy, remains to be established. The apparent association with high foetal mortality is very questionable. Until these aspects are clarified by further studies no firm guidelines on management of patients with widespread prurigo can be given. It is certainly no longer applicable to prescribe diethylstilboestrol as its use in pregnancy has been associated with development of vaginal adenocarcinomata in the offspring.

PRURITIC FOLLICULITIS OF PREGNANCY

Clinical features   Although few cases of this disorder have been published, mild forms of the eruption are probably not uncommon. It consists of erythematous follicular papules and pustules (Fig. 17.3) usually widely distributed. The onset is from 4–9 months gestation and resolution from 5 months gestation to 1 month post-partum. The foetal and maternal prognoses are normal. The cause remains unknown.

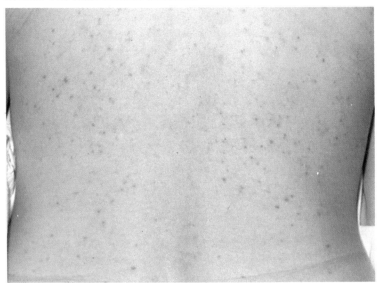

Fig. 17.3   Pruritic folliculitis of pregnancy—follicular lesions on the back.

PEMPHIGOID GESTATIONIS (HERPES GESTATIONIS)

Clinical features   Pemphigoid gestationis (PG) is a bullous disease principally associated with pregnancy but may also occur with trophoblastic tumours. PG is closely related, clinically and pathologically, to the pemphigoid group of disorders. The title 'pemphigoid gestationis' is therefore to be preferred to its old misleading name. While PG is very rare, occurring in as few as 1 in 60 000 pregnancies, the diagnosis is frequently considered because of the clinical overlap with the much more common eruption PEP. They are now recognized as distinct: useful differentiating features are listed in Table 17.2. Both PG and PEP may exhibit erythematous papules, target lesions and vesicles: however, only in PG do the patients develop large tense bullae (Fig. 17.4).

Management   Treatment of PG depends upon its severity. In the early stages and in mild cases adequate symptomatic control may be achieved with a topical corticosteroid cream but, in more florid cases, systemic corticosteroids are needed. It usually settles promptly with 40 mg of prednisolone daily and the dose may then be reduced to the minimum. This varies throughout

Table 17.2 Differentiating features of polymorphic eruption of pregnancy (PEP) and pemphigoid gestationis (PG)

	PEP	PG
Primiparous	80%	50%
Morphology		
Erythematous papules	+	+
Target lesions	+	+
Vesicles	+	+
Bullae	−	+
Prominent striae	+	−
Periumbilical lesions	−	+
Foetal prognosis	Normal	Impaired
Recurrence in subsequent pregnancies	−	+
Immunofluorescence for C_3 at the BMZ		
Direct IMF (skin)	−	100%
Indirect IMF (serum)	−	80%
HLA associations	−	A1, B8, DR3
Associated autoimmune phenomena (e.g. Graves' disease)	−	+

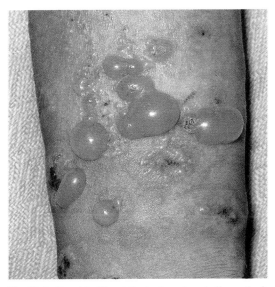

Fig. 17.4 Pemphigoid gestationis—large tense bullae on the forearm.

pregnancy so that close monitoring of the patient's clinical progress is necessary. The dose of prednisolone needed often falls sharply towards the end of pregnancy but invariably rises briskly immediately after delivery. The duration of treatment needed post-partum varies from a few weeks to several years. Prednisolone in the doses outlined in the second and third trimesters does not appear to affect the foetus.

Where systemic corticosteroids are contraindicated, plasmapheresis should be considered. It is equally effective whether fresh frozen plasma or purified protein derivative is used.

Vital to the management of PG is close supervision of the foetal progress. PG can be associated with impaired placental function and there is a significant increase in the frequency of small-for-dates infants. Foetal distress may lead to Caesarian section in some cases and more frequently the infants have to be admitted to special care baby units. Patients with PG should be delivered only in maternity units with facilities for intensive care of the newborn. After delivery, patients should be warned that the eruption will almost certainly recur in all further pregnancies and is likely to be more severe. They should also avoid taking oral contraceptives as they may induce a recurrence.

In PG there is an increase in the frequency of the HLA haplotype A1, B8, DR3 which is associated with autoimmune phenomena. An association between PG and Graves' disease has been described. When managing PG, therefore, the possibility of coexistent autoimmune disorders should be considered.

PUSTULAR PSORIASIS OF PREGNANCY (IMPETIGO HERPETIFORMIS)

Clinical features
This eruption was initially considered (by Hebra) to be specifically related to pregnancy but it has since been described in non-pregnant women and in men. It is now regarded as an exanthematic form of pustular psoriasis. How pregnancy can precipitate this eruption in latent psoriatics is not clear. It may be secondary to the rise in progesterone during pregnancy, as giving progesterone to non-pregnant women has been associated with the onset of severe pustular psoriasis.

Management
In addition to their eruption, patients frequently develop fever, delirium, diarrhoea and vomiting. The management of the condition is an acute medical emergency. Without urgent correction of the dehydration and electrolyte disturbance, there is a high maternal and foetal mortality.

In addition to the correction of their metabolic disturbances, prednisolone 15–30 mg daily is often effective in controlling the eruption. Antibiotics are indicated on evidence of secondary bacterial infection.

Patients with pustular psoriasis in pregnancy should be advised against further pregnancies as the eruption may recur.

FURTHER READING

Holmes R C, Black M M 1982 The specific dermatoses of pregnancy. Journal of the American Academy of Dermatology 8: 405–412
Winton G B, Lewis C W 1982 Dermatoses of pregnancy. Journal of the American Academy of Dermatology 6: 977–998

R. A. Marsden

18. Bullous Dermatoses

Accurate diagnosis of the bullous diseases and, ultimately, their successful management, depends largely upon the histology and direct immunofluorescence (IMF) findings which, in turn, depend on the quality of specimens submitted to the laboratory for examination. All biopsies must be taken by an experienced clinician and lesions selected for histology must be less than 24 hours old. Fresh or snap-frozen peri-lesional or uninvolved skin should be sent to the laboratory immediately for direct IMF. If this is not possible, buffered transport medium will preserve the tissue for several days.

PEMPHIGUS

Clinical features   Pemphigus is a group of disorders with keratinocyte separation (acantholysis) and intradermal blister formation. There are IgG deposits between epidermal cells on direct IMF in virtually every patient with active disease and circulating IgG antibody against epidermal intercellular substance can be detected in over 90% of cases.

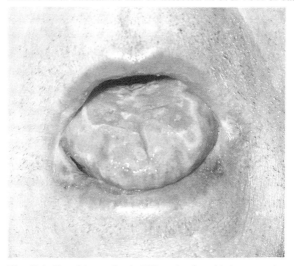

Fig. 18.1 Pemphigus vulgaris. This patient's oral lesions caused considerable distress and were unresponsive to high doses of prednisolone and chlorambucil.

Pemphigus vulgaris

Oral lesions usually appear first (Fig. 18.1), to be followed weeks or months later by thin roofed, flaccid supra basal blisters on the skin which rupture to leave painful, bleeding and crusted erosions. The skin is often extremely fragile and may blister with relatively minor friction injury.

The disease was invariably fatal in the pre-steroid era. However, the prognosis has gradually improved and with steroid-sparing drugs, over 50% of patients can be expected to achieve complete remission. Most deaths are attributable to the complications of treatment, the commonest being pneumonia or septicaemia, and not unexpectedly most occur in the elderly. Estimating serum antibody titres and serial skin biopsies for direct IMF are rough guides to disease activity. Loss of antibody from the skin or blood is usually a favourable prognostic signal though caution is needed. In the final analysis, the decision to reduce the dose of prednisolone or to stop treatment is a clinical one.

Pemphigus vegetans

This is a chronic variant of pemphigus vulgaris with vegetations at lip margins and in the flexures. The prognosis is better than that of pemphigus vulgaris.

Pemphigus foliaceus

Pemphigus foliaceus is more benign than pemphigus vulgaris. There are more superficial sub-corneal blisters with scaling crusted lesions predominantly on the scalp, face or upper chest (Fig. 18.2). Flaccid

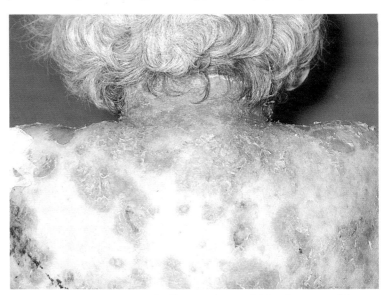

Fig. 18.2 Pemphigus foliaceus. This illustrates the superficial scaling nature of the disorder.

blisters may form particularly at the edge of spreading lesions. Oral involvement is uncommon. The IMF findings in most patients are identical to those of pemphigus vulgaris with intercellular IgG deposited through the full thickness of the epidermis. In some cases the IgG may be confined to the superficial epidermis.

Management   When the diagnosis has been established the patient and relatives should be warned of the serious nature of the illness and the need for rigorous treatment explained. Pemphigus should whenever possible be treated on an out-patient basis with its lower risk of infection.

If hospital care is necessary, the patient should be reverse barrier nursed in a single ward. The patient with extensive lesions should be nursed on an absorbent, non-adherent sheet on a ripple bed or better still on an air bed.

Bacteriological swabs should be taken regularly from skin, mouth and eyes, and secondary infection treated with the appropriate antibiotic. *Staphylococcus aureus* is the commonest pathogen, for which prophylactic flucloxacillin 1.5–2 g daily is recommended. Suitable local antiseptics include 0.5% acetic acid, 0.5% silver nitrate solution, silver sulphadiazine cream 1%, all of which are active against pseudomonas, or gentian violet or potassium permanganate solutions for weeping or flexural areas.

Tight dressings, tape and bandages can induce skin lesions, so should be avoided if possible. A non-adherent dressing such as paraffin gauze can be applied to areas needing protection. A potent topical steroid cream, e.g. 0.05% clobetasol propionate, can be applied directly to erosions.

Fortunately, most pemphigus vulgaris presents with oral lesions or with relatively localized skin disease. In these cases, 40 mg of prednisolone taken on alternate mornings with azathioprine 100–150 mg daily is usually effective and well tolerated. Treatment should continue for about 12 months after skin healing, and the dose of prednisolone should be reduced slowly. After a further 12 months the azathioprine can be withdrawn. There may be late recurrences and so prolonged follow-up is desirable. Patients failing to respond or patients with extensive life-threatening disease need more aggressive therapy and should be given 150–200 mg daily of prednisolone in addition to azathioprine. If there is no improvement in 5–10 days the dose of prednisolone should be doubled to 300–400 mg daily. The dose of prednisolone can be halved once the skin has healed (a falling antibody titre is also encouraging) then reduced over the following 3 weeks to be maintained at 40 mg on alternate mornings. If the disease recurs the prednisolone dose should be increased temporarily.

Therapy is empirical. Controlled trials have not been carried out in pemphigus. The addition of a steroid sparing agent, e.g. azathioprine undoubtedly improves disease control and prognosis. Alternatives to azathioprine are methotrexate, cyclophosphamide, gold and dapsone. Prednisolone, azathioprine and gold can be combined for severe cases and a fourth drug added if control is not rapid. The value of plasmapheresis or plasma exchange in pemphigus vulgaris is as yet unproven but may be justified in desperate cases.

Oral lesions are painful, demoralising and can persist for many months after skin healing. Their continued presence should not prevent the reduction of the prednisolone dose when the skin has cleared. The following regimen is recommended: a 0.5 mg tablet of betamethasone phosphate is dissolved in 5 ml of water and the solution rinsed vigorously around the mouth for 5 minutes before spitting out. The contents of a capsule containing tetracycline 250 mg and nystatin 250 000 units are then suspended in 5 ml of water, rinsed around the mouth for 5 minutes and then spat out. The treatment is repeated at 6-hourly invervals.

Stubborn lesions can be treated with triamcinolone in adhesive base or by injections of triamcinolone suspension into the base of an ulcer. The lips can be treated with a potent steroid ointment. Secondary infection with candida and Vincent's organisms is common. The former can be treated with amphotericin lozenges, the latter with metronidazole tablets.

Pemphigus foliaceus
Mild pemphigus and pemphigus erythematodes (Senear-Usher disease) may be well controlled by topical clobetasol propionate alone. In more severe disease, systemic prednisolone and a steroid sparing agent may be necessary. The case management is similar to that of pemphigus vulgaris.

BULLOUS PEMPHIGOID

Clinical features
In bullous pemphigoid, large tense subepidermal blisters appear on a background of normal or pruritic erythematous skin (Fig. 18.3). The diagnosis is confirmed by direct IMF which shows a linear band of IgG and/or C3 at the dermo-epidermal junction of perilesional or uninvolved skin. There may be a circulating antibasement membrane zone (BMZ) antibody in up to 80% of active cases shown by indirect IMF techniques

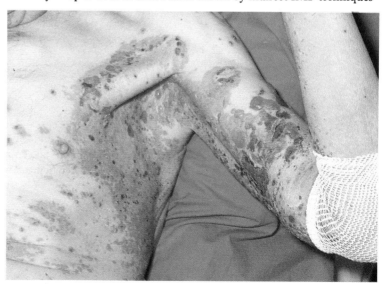

Fig. 18.3 Bullous pemphigoid. Tense, haemorrhagic blisters present.

although titres show no relationship to the severity of disease. Most patients with bullous pemphigoid are elderly, though it can occur in younger persons and even in children. The death rate varies from 6–36%, patients succumbing mainly from treatment side-effects or from unrelated causes.

Management   Most patients with bullous pemphigoid can be nursed in an ordinary bed. The lesions are dressed with paraffin gauze, antiseptics or a very potent topical steroid.

No controlled therapeutic trials have been carried out. Most patients with bullous pemphigoid are given and respond to 60–100 mg prednisolone daily. Only in rare cases are higher doses necessary. Indeed patients of 80 years or more, or with relatively localized disease, may respond to 20–30 mg prednisolone daily. Azathioprine 1.5 mg per kilogram body weight can be started at the same time as it is well tolerated. It may avoid some of the more serious side effects of corticosteroid therapy and shorten treatment. With the disease under control the dose of prednisolone can be reduced over several weeks to 10–15 mg daily. Elderly patients may not cope with alternate day regimens. Every 6 months an attempt to discontinue therapy should be made as most patients surviving the first 12 weeks of treatment eventually achieve full remission.

Long acting tetracosactrin 2 mg intramuscularly twice weekly for 2 weeks, then 1 mg intramuscularly twice weekly for 2 weeks, is a suitable alternative to higher doses of prednisolone for frail or elderly patients. The tetracosactrin is eventually replaced by maintenance doses of prednisolone 10–15 mg daily. Dapsone and sulphapyridine may be effective in bullous pemphigoid, particularly adults under 60 years of age, children, or where the histology shows a neutrophil rather than an eosinophil infiltrate.

CICATRICIAL PEMPHIGOID (BENIGN MUCOUS MEMBRANE PEMPHIGOID)

Clinical features   Cicatricial pemphigoid is uncommon, seen mainly in the elderly. It features recurrent blistering and scarring of the mucous membranes, mainly the conjunctivae, mouth and skin. Ocular complications include synechiae*, symblepharon* and entropion; in advanced cases there may be keratitis, corneal ulceration and blindness. Skin lesions are usually quite localized with a tendency to recur at the same site. Direct and indirect IMF findings may be similar to those of bullous pemphigoid but fewer than 50% of patients give positive results.

Management   There is no consistently effective treatment for cicatricial pemphigoid. Systemic treatment with prednisolone and azathioprine may be indicated for a widespread rash or for oesophageal and laryngeal lesions. Dapsone

*Synechia, an adhesion formed between the iris and the posterior surface of the cornea, or the anterior capsule of the lens.
*Symblepharon, adhesion of the eyelid to the eyeball.

may also be effective. Skin lesions often respond to a potent topical steroid or intralesional triamcinolone.

DERMATITIS HERPETIFORMIS

Clinical features   The intensely pruritic papulo-vesicular eruption of dermatitis herpetiformis occurs predominantly on the face, scalp, shoulders, buttocks and extensor aspect of the limbs. Scratching soon damages the vesicles so that in many cases excoriations are the most prominent clinical feature. The diagnosis is confirmed by histology, with sub-epidermal vesicle formation and neutrophil microabscesses in adjacent dermal papillae and by direct IMF showing granular deposition of IgA in the papillary dermis. Most patients, if not all, show evidence of coeliac disease on jejunal biopsy. Frank malabsorption, however, is uncommon except in children, where gastrointestinal symptoms may precede the rash by many years. As in coeliac disease, the incidence of HLAB8 and DR3 is raised. The disease has a prolonged course, although spontaneous remissions can occur which, in about 10% of cases, may be permanent.

Management   Dapsone, the treatment of choice, produces dramatic relief from pruritus within 24 hours and stops new lesion formation within 72 hours. When dapsone is discontinued, lesions tend to reappear within 3–7 days. Most respond to an initial dose of 100 mg daily but some may need up to 400 mg daily. After the skin has cleared, the optimum maintenance dose, i.e. the smallest dose to keep the patient free or virtually free of lesions, should then be found. Doses as low as 50 mg once or twice weekly may be effective.

The commonest side effects of dapsone are methaemoglobinaemia and haemolysis. Fortunately, both tend to be mild and are usually symptomatic. The former is an idiosyncratic reaction, possibly dependent on the patient's acetylator status while the latter is dose dependent. Both are more severe in children and the elderly.

Other dapsone side effects include headache, peripheral neuropathy and agranulocytosis, which are rare, and the latter potentially lethal. The dapsone hypersensitivity syndrome, usually in the fifth or sixth week of therapy, features a rash, hepatitis, albuminuria, lymphadenopathy and leucopenia. Regular blood checks are advised for patients with dermatitis herpetiformis receiving long term dapsone therapy.

Alternatives to dapsone: people intolerant to dapsone might be given sulphapyridine 0.25–3 g daily, 2 g being the approximate therapeutic equivalent of 100 mg of dapsone. In Britain the drug is still available from the manufacturer on a named-patient basis.

Sulphamethoxypyridiazine is a long-acting sulphonamide, 1 g being equivalent to 100 mg of dapsone. The effective dose varies from 0.5–1.0 gm daily. Side effects, mostly cutaneous, are more common with doses greater than 1 gm daily. Oral sodium cromoglycate, heparin, indomethacin and cholestyramine are also reported to be effective in dermatitis herpetiformis, but in practice are rarely needed.

Gluten-free diet   All patients with dermatitis herpetiformis, including those with an apparently normal jejunal biopsy should take a strict gluten-free diet under the supervision of an experienced dietician. Patients should also join coeliac societies which provide detailed and up-to-date information on gluten in manufactured foods. However, the difficulties of such a diet may not make it feasible in people of low intelligence, the elderly, persons living alone who cook for themselves, or those who have to eat in canteens, restaurants etc. Many patients with dermatitis herpetiformis are able to discontinue drug therapy after 6 months to 9 years on a gluten-free diet. A gluten-free diet also helps improve the general condition and increase the sense of well-being of patients with gastrointestinal symptoms due to malabsorption and some with apparently asymptomatic coeliac disease. A gluten-free diet may provide some protection from gastrointestinal lymphoma and carcinoma which have increased incidences in dermatitis herpetiformis.

LINEAR IgA DERMATOSIS OF CHILDHOOD (CHRONIC BULLOUS DERMATOSIS OF CHILDHOOD)

Clinical features   Linear IgA disease of childhood is a vesiculo-bullous, pemphigoid-like disorder but characterized by deposition of IgA in a linear band along the basement membrane. Its relationship to linear IgA disease of adults is uncertain. It tends to remit spontaneously after several years but may persist into adult life.

Management   Most patients respond to sulphapyridine or dapsone. Begin with 1–2 g of sulphapyridine daily, increasing to 2–3 g daily after 7 days if not significantly improved. If this is unhelpful, substitute dapsone 50–150 mg daily or sulphamethoxypyridiazine 1–1.5 g daily. Unfortunately neither dapsone, sulphapyridine, nor sulphamethoxypyridiazine are available in liquid form. Tablets can be crushed and mixed with jam or honey to mask the taste. In refractory cases, prednisolone, initial dose 20–30 mg daily, may be needed. Conjunctival involvement and scarring, sometimes asymptomatic, occur in patients with long-standing disease, so that regular ophthalmological examination is always indicated.

LINEAR IgA DERMATOSIS OF ADULTS

Clinical features   Most patients have a rash indistinguishable from dermatitis herpetiformis but some have features more suggestive of bullous pemphigoid.

Management   Most respond well to dapsone therapy alone. However, some need a combination of dapsone 50–100 mg daily and prednisolone, doses ranging from 5–20 mg daily.

CHRONIC BENIGN FAMILIAL PEMPHIGUS (HAILEY-HAILEY DISEASE)

Clinical features

This is an uncommon chronic, genodermatosis of autosomal dominant inheritance usually beginning in the 15–30 age group, characterized by vesiculation, exudation, crusting and fissuring of the neck, genitalia and body folds (Fig. 18.4). Oral and oesophageal lesions have been reported. Exacerbations are precipitated by heat, trauma, ultra-violet light and bacterial and candidal infection. The histological hallmark is acantholysis with partial cell separation giving the appearance of a dilapidated brick wall. Direct IMF of the skin is negative.

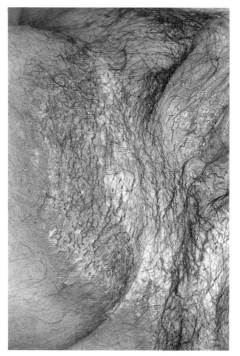

Fig. 18.4   Hailey-Hailey disease. Fissured exudative lesions in the groin.

Management

The response to treatment is unpredictable and usually temporary. Aggravating factors such as excessive friction, sunlight, heat and obesity must be avoided. Bacteriological swabs should be taken regularly and the appropriate oral antimicrobial given. A topical steroid/antibacterial or anti-candidal preparation may be effective and is worth trying before considering other options such as Grenz rays or excision of the affected areas followed by split skin grafting. The latter may work simply by reducing the number of sweat glands and therefore the amount of sweating in flexural areas. It may bring long-term benefit, although lesions may continue to appear within and around the grafted areas.

FURTHER READING

Fry L et al 1982 Long term follow up of dermatitis herpetiformis with and without dietary gluten withdrawal. British Journal of Dermatology 107: 631–640

Levene G M 1982 The treatment of pemphigus and pemphigoid. Clinical and Experimental Dermatology 7: 643–652

Lever W F, Schaumburg-Lever G 1984 Treatment of pemphigus vulgaris. Results obtained in 4 patients between 1961 and 1982. Archives of Dermatology 120: 44–47

Marsden R A 1982 The treatment of benign chronic bullous dermatosis of childhood, and dermatitis herpetiformis and bullous pemphigoid beginning in childhood. Clinical and Experimental Dermatology 7: 653–663

Savin J A 1981 Some factors affecting prognosis in pemphigus vulgaris and pemphigoid. British Journal of Dermatology 104: 415–420

W. R. Tyldesley

19. Dermatoses with Oral Involvement

Management of oral mucosal lesions depends greatly on the use of non-specific therapy to reduce secondary infection and, hence, pain and discomfort. A much more satisfactory environment may then be achieved for the use of any available specific measures.

GENERAL THERAPY

Covering agents

Adhesive substances such as carboxymethylcellulose paste may provide more or less substantial protection for an ulcerated or erosive lesion by their simple covering action. They are not particularly easy to use nor very retentive but may prove useful in relatively restricted minor lesions. They may also be used as vehicles for more active therapy such as anti-inflammatory agents, corticosteroids and antifungals.

Antiseptic mouthwashes

Many proprietary preparations may help to reduce the discomfort of minor oral lesions. No one product is clearly superior to the others in general but the binding of chlorhexidine to the oral mucosa makes it particularly useful. Chlorhexidine, by reducing the rate of formation of dental plaque, is valuable when mucosal instability makes oral hygiene difficult to maintain.

Antibiotics and antifungals

In more widely erosive lesions, antibiotic mouthwashes may give dramatic relief. Tetracyclines are most often used—2% chlortetracycline as a mouthwash with 10% glycerol is particularly useful in reducing secondary infection and, therefore, discomfort in many conditions. For example, in acute herpetic stomatitis, the pain and discomfort are often rapidly relieved by such a mouthwash—the same tetracycline given systemically may have much less effect. In a few conditions these agents appear to be specific, for instance, the rapid response of the herpetiform variant of recurrent oral ulceration to tetracycline mouthwashes is virtually diagnostic. Problems with atrophic candidosis may occur but they are much less frequent than might be expected, even with prolonged courses. The often quoted advice to restrict such courses to 5 days seems unnecessary. If problems arise (or are anticipated in an at-risk patient) a locally-acting antifungal such as an imidazole should be added.

Antibiotic ointments and creams may help lesions of the lips, particularly angular cheilitis and fissures. It is often difficult to assess, clinically, whether candida or staphylococci are involved. If candida are present then amphotericin B cream is commonly used; if staphylococci, fucidic acid cream. If both are involved, or if bacteriological confirmation is not available, miconazole cream with its combined antibacterial and antifungal action, is valuable. A similar approach is made to denture stomatitis; creams may conveniently be applied on the fitting surface of dentures.

In immunologically-compromised patients, bacterial plaque-like lesions may occur on the oral mucosa or lips (Fig. 19.1). Often simulating herpes or thrush, they may be populated by almost pure strains of

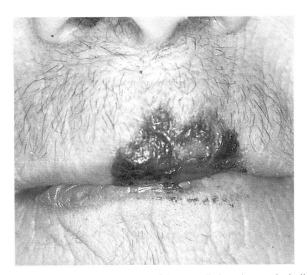

Fig. 19.1 Staphylococcal lesion of the upper lip in an immunologically compromised patient rapidly responsive to local and systemic penicillin.

organisms which in other circumstances are considered non-pathogens. Local and systemic antibiotics are used, the choice depending entirely on the identification and sensitivity testing of the organism. If a suitable locally-acting preparation is not available, one should be improvised for the specific circumstances. Trypsinization is also used to disintegrate the mucoid matrix of the lesions.

Anaesthetic preparations

In erosive or ulcerative conditions of the oral mucosa, eating may be painful or even virtually impossible. Lozenges, sprays and mouthwashes containing local anaesthetics may help. A lignocaine mouthwash is particularly useful and can be prepared conveniently by diluting lignocaine viscous preparations to a final concentration of 0.5%. In isolated painful lesions of the mucosa lignocaine ointment may help, although it is often difficult to apply and to retain.

Moisturizing mouthwashes

'Dry mouth' of whatever origin may improve with moisturizing mouthwashes containing either glycerol or methylcellulose. Trials have not shown any distinct advantage of one over the other and neither is, in fact, particularly useful as the effect is relatively transient. There is no known practical way of stimulating salivary flow in patients with partial salivary gland degeneration. Many dry mouths are drug-induced and so, at least in theory, reversible by drug change or withdrawal.

Mucolytic agents

When stasis in the mouth leads to plaque-like deposits (particularly on the tongue) a mucolytic agent reduces the adherence and density of the coating. Ascorbic acid mouthwashes do this. When adherent infective plaques form on the oral mucosa, as may occur in immunologically compromised patients, trypsinization may (in combination with antibiotic therapy) bring about distintegration of the lesions.

Surgery

Laser surgery and cryosurgery are advocated for the treatment of persistent oral lesions. Their limitations in chronic and recurrent conditions such as major erosive lichen planus are obvious. Clearly, however, it may be the choice in oral lesions (such as leukoplakia) which are more local.

Corticosteroids

When the mouth is involved in a severe, generalized steroid-sensitive disease, systemic steroids may be needed, with steroid-sparing drugs if indicated. Dosages which suppress oral lesions may need to be high—in many conditions oral lesions are less responsive than those of the skin or of other mucous membranes. However, in most conditions in which oral lesions predominate, systemic steroids may be replaced by local therapy in a wide dose range. Specifically-designed oral preparations are relatively few and of low potency (hydrocortisone lozenges, 2.5 mg are an example) but may help such conditions as minor aphthous ulceration. Steroids in adhesive bases may be useful for relatively isolated lesions in accessible areas but are difficult to apply. Steroid metered aerosol sprays (as for asthma) may be used on inaccessible sites such as the soft palate.

For more aggressive therapy, individually prepared mouthwashes including known amounts of steroid in relatively high concentration should be used. This is a technique which can reduce the incidence of steroid-induced side-effects, although they may not be entirely eliminated as there may be significant absorption. Prednisolone, betamethasone, triamcinolone or other steroids are used in this way. For example, triamcinolone is helpful in daily totals of 0.75 mg, 1.5 mg, 3 mg (or, occasionally, considerably more) using a 2% chlortetracycline mouthwash as a vehicle. Each application must be measured accurately in a way not usual with mouthwashes. Steroid creams and ointments may be used on the lips. With significant lesions, such as major erosive lichen planus, more powerful preparations than 1% hydrocortisone are needed.

SPECIFIC MEASURES FOR THE MANAGEMENT OF ORAL LESIONS

Angular cheilitis

Identify and correct any possible precipitating factor—ill-fitting dentures, anaemias etc. Swabs should be used to determine an infective component, usually candida and/or staphylococci. They should be treated accordingly with local preparations. Angular cheilitis in Crohn's disease or eczema responds to 1% hydrocortisone.

Erythema multiforme

This is often restricted to the mouth with no obvious precipitating factor. It usually affects the lower lip (Fig. 19.2). In these circumstances triamcinolone and chlortetracycline mouthwashes should be used. If other areas are significantly involved, systemic steroids in short reducing courses and systemic antibiotics are indicated.

Glossitis (midline)

The condition is not, as previously thought, a developmental lesion but a form of chronic candidosis (Fig. 19.3). An imidazole oral gel should be used for a protracted period.

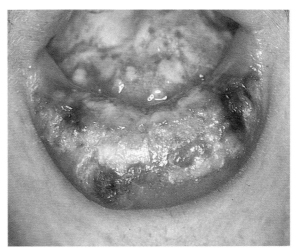

Fig. 19.2 Erythema multiforme restricted to the mouth. The involvement of the lower lip is characteristic.

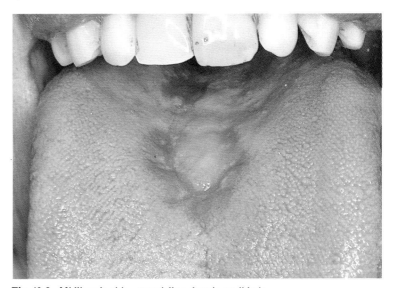

Fig. 19.3 Midline glossitis—essentially a chronic candidosis.

Leukoplakia (Fig. 19.4)

Management is predominantly surgical and depends on histological assessment. If candida is involved, an imidazole should be used followed by surgery; cryosurgery is often very effective.

Lichen planus

If non erosive, this is symptom-free and unresponsive to any form of treatment (see Ch. 11).

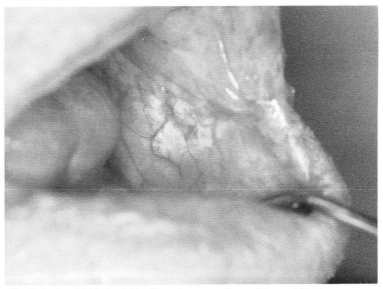

Fig. 19.4 Candidal leukoplakia of buccal mucosa—the candida are within the epithelium.

In the minor erosive form, betamethasone-17-valerate metered aerosol or beclomethasone, 17,21 dipropionate metered aerosol should be used together with chlorhexidine mouthwashes.

In the major erosive form, triamcinolone-chlortetracycline mouthwashes may give control but this is a resistant condition. Lignocaine mouthwashes may be used for comfort.

Pemphigoid (mucosal or generalized) (see Ch. 18)

Betamethasone-17-valerate metered aerosol or beclomethasone, 17,21 dipropionate metered aerosol will control bulla formation. Chlorhexidine mouthwashes reduce the discomfort of ruptured bullae. In more severe cases triamcinolone-chlortetracycline mouthwashes are recommended.

Pemphigus vulgaris (see Ch. 18)

Oral lesions may remain after the skin lesions are under control. High concentrations of triamcinolone-chlortetracycline and lignocaine mouthwashes should be used in addition to systemic therapy.

Recurrent oral ulceration

Any possible aetiological factor such as flat jejunal mucosa, folate, vitamin B_{12} or iron deficiency should be determined. If detected this should be corrected. Approximately 6% of all patients have such an aetiology.

For minor aphthous ulceration simple covering agents, chlorhexidine mouthwashes, hydrocortisone pellets or triamcinolone paste should be used.

In major aphthous ulceration (Fig. 19.5), triamcinolone-chlortetracycline and lignocaine mouthwashes are used. Where this is part of Bechcet's syndrome this should be treated in the same way unless other system involvement necessitates systemic treatment.

Herpetiform ulceration is most often associated with nutritional abnormality. It is not steroid responsive but highly responsive to local (not systemic) tetracyclines. In spite of its name it is not due to herpes virus.

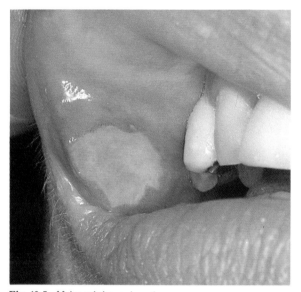

Fig. 19.5   Major aphthous ulceration.

Sjögren's (Sicca) syndrome

'Dry mouth' is very difficult to treat. Moisturizing mouthwashes are of transient value only. No method is available to increase salivary flow.

Crohn's disease (see Ch. 12)

FURTHER READING

Tyldesley W R 1981 Oral medicine. Oxford University Press, Oxford

S. M. Burge and R. P. R. Dawber

20. Dermatoses Involving the Hair and Nails

HAIR

The growing hair follicle consists of an outer root sheath, continuous with the overlying epidermis, a specialized inner root sheath, a germinal zone (matrix) around the dermal papilla and a central developing hair (Fig. 20.1). The root sheaths mould the hair shaft growing within it.

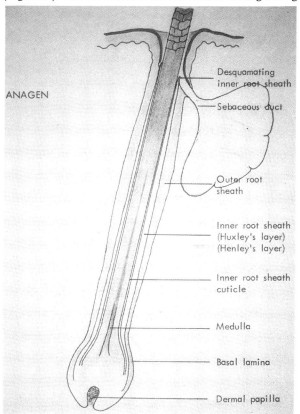

Fig. 20.1 Fully developed anagen (growing) follicle with emerging hair.

Each hair follicle undergoes repeated cycles of growth and rest. During the anagen (growing) phase, the lower part of the follicle partially encloses the dermal papilla, which consists of specialized cells important in controlling the activity of hair bulb matrix cells. The matrix cells proliferate to form the inner root sheath and hair shaft. Every 3–6 years anagen ceases, mitosis in the matrix decreases, the inner root sheath disappears and the follicle gradually shortens (catagen phase). The follicle then enters the resting or telogen phase during which normal telogen shedding occurs (Fig. 20.2). The follicle re-enters anagen spontaneously or may be induced to do so by plucking. The new hair grows up alongside the resting telogen (club) hair. In the normal scalp at least 80% of follicles are in anagen.

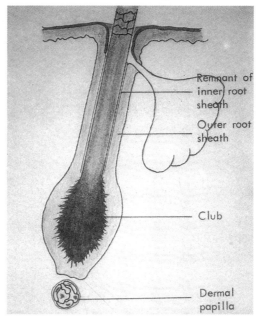

Fig. 20.2   Club hair in a shortened telogen (resting) follicle.

HIRSUTISM

Clinical features   Hirsutism is growth in the female of terminal (coarse) hair partly or wholly in the adult male pattern, induced by androgenic stimulation.

Management   Adrenal or ovarian pathology must be excluded and the following considered:
1.   Age of onset and racial factors. Mild hirsutism is normal in some cases
2.   Menstrual history and fertility
3.   Weight variations: obesity is one sign of the polycystic ovary syndrome. Weight loss due to anorexia may be associated with hirsutism.
4.   Signs of virilization, e.g. cliteromegaly
5.   Presence of other androgen related cutaneous disease, e.g. diffuse alopecia, acne

6. Serum testosterone and sex hormone binding globulin should be measured. Full androgen assessment is unnecessary in patients with normal testosterone levels and regular menstrual cycles (Rentoul et al).

A fertile woman with a regular menstrual cycle and mild hirsutism commencing after puberty is unlikely to have a serious disorder. The patient should be re-assured if there is no serious abnormality and appropriate measures may include:
1. Bleaching
2. Shaving, waxing, plucking or chemical hair removers. Plucking synchronizes the production of hairs by the plucked follicles but does not increase the number of hairs produced
3. Electrolysis is the only practical permanent procedure. Treatment is limited by cost and time. 25–100 hairs can be removed per treatment but up to 40%, depending on the skill of the electrolysis, will regrow because the bulb is not destroyed
4. Systemic anti-androgens (such as cyproterone acetate). Unfortunately hirsutism takes up to a year to improve and facial hair is the most resistant to treatment.

COMMON BALDNESS

Clinical features   Common or androgenic baldness is normal in men and in many women from puberty onwards. Genetically predisposed terminal follicles on the vertex of the scalp are converted to vellus type by androgen.

In males the baldness is patterned with severity ranging from mild bitemporal recession or vertex loss to confluent loss, sparing the posterior, and lateral scalp margins. Most affected females have slightly raised androgen levels, combined with a familial tendency to baldness. Other androgen dependent conditions may be present, e.g. hirsutism and acne. The hair loss is diffuse and rarely progresses to complete baldness. Other causes of diffuse loss must be excluded (see below).

Management   The patient must be given a full explanation of the significance of the hair loss and helped to come to terms with it. Those with personality problems may relate their inadequacies to the hair loss but will not find life any simpler with a full head of hair. In a few men, hair transplantation may be considered but it is expensive, results are variable and patients with inadequate personalities will be no better off. A wig may be the best approach in women with extensive diffuse loss.

Most patients with diffuse hair loss have physiological androgenic alopecia. Some have an abnormal psychological reaction to a mild degree of hair thinning and may require long-term emotional support.

There is a suicide risk in the more severely affected patient. It may be necessary to enlist the help of the general practitioner, social worker or psychiatrist for those who 'magnify' the hair loss—the so-called dysmorphophobic group.

The antihypertensive, minoxidil, causes regrowth when given orally but cannot be used in normotensive individuals. Its use topically has not been proven to be effective. The antiandrogen, cyproterone acetate, has been used systemically in females to reverse or halt androgen induced cutaneous disease, e.g. acne vulgaris, diffuse alopecia, hirsutism. The cyproterone is administered with an oestrogen, ethinyloestradiol, in a contraceptive pill (cyproterone acetate 2 mg, ethinyloestradiol 0.05 mg). The pill is taken from day 5 to day 25 of the menstrual cycle. In most cases it is necessary to use additional cyproterone acetate (50–100 mg/day). Oestrogens are always given with anti-androgens to prevent pregnancy, since cyproterone acetate may cause profound fetal abnormalities and feminization of a male fetus.

Treatment of alopecia must last 18 months to 2 years. The rate of telogen shedding is reduced (this can be monitored with serial telogen counts from the vertex); the shaft diameter of remaining terminal hairs increase and the reduced greasiness improves the texture of the hair. Unfortunately, there is very little regrowth of terminal hair from follicles which have become vellus.

Side-effects are most likely in the first 3 months of treatment with anti-androgens but gradually lessen: dysmenorrhoea, breast tenderness and decreased libido are common. Thrombophlebitis may occur and hepatitis is a rare complication. Liver function tests should be monitored. A barrier form of contraceptive should be used for the first 3 months until treatment is established.

As with contraceptive pills, contraindications include obesity, hypertension, smoking, thrombophlebitis, older patients.

CHRONIC DIFFUSE ALOPECIA

Clinical features   A diffuse, non-scarring alopecia may be associated with several underlying disorders:
1. Hypothyroidism
2. Nutritional deficiencies
    a. Essential fatty acid deficiency, e.g. patients receiving chronic parenteral nutrition.
    b. Zinc deficiency, e.g. patients receiving chronic parenteral nutrition, alcoholism; children with acrodermatitis enteropathica (unable to absorb zinc).
    c. Iron deficiency.
    d. Malabsorption.
3. Drugs
    a. Anticoagulants, e.g. heparin and warfarin.
    b. Cytostatics.

Management   Treatment is of the underlying cause. This may result in regrowth but in hypothyroidism and iron deficiency results may be disappointing.

TELOGEN EFFLUVIUM

Clinical features   3–4 months after stress, iron deficiency, fever, haemorrhage, 'crash' dieting, telogen effluvium may be precipitated. In this, most of the follicles pass into telogen. It is always diffuse and very rarely total.

Post partum hair loss is a form of telogen effluvium. The percentage of hair in anagen increases to about 95% during pregnancy so that normal telogen shedding is reduced. After parturition (oestrogen decrease) these follicles rapidly enter catagen and then telogen, resulting in increased shedding three to four months later. This continues for several months. Further telogen loss may be due to blood loss and stress.

Management   No treatment is required other than reassurance as spontaneous regrowth occurs over the next 6 months.

ALOPECIA AREATA

Clinical features   The initial lesion is characteristically a well demarcated, totally bald, smooth, white patch of skin, which is found by chance. The diagnosis is confirmed by finding broken 'exclamation mark' hairs (Fig. 20.3) in a normal scalp. Bad prognostic factors include associated atopic disease, repeated attacks or extensive loss.

Numerous 'moth eaten' areas of patchy loss may be due to secondary syphilis which should be excluded. In chronic lesions it may be difficult to exclude scarring alopecia and biopsy is sometimes necessary. In children, trichotillomania may simulate alopecia areata.

Management   The unpredictable nature of the disease should be explained to the patient. Emotional support must be provided and a wig may be required. Unfortunately, no treatments alter the long-term prognosis.

Circumscribed alopecia has a good prognosis and treatment is unnecessary.

Systemic corticosteroids restore temporary hair growth in the majority of patients but the dose required may produce serious side-effects. Topical steroids do not help. Intralesional steroids can promote regrowth over a limited area, such as the eyebrows, but atrophy is a potential complication.

Temporary regrowth may be induced by treatment with dinitrochlorobenzene (DNCB) and squaric acid dibutylester (SADBE) applied locally to induce contact dermatitis (possibly by alteration in immunoregulation). DNCB is mutagenic and possibly carcinogenic, so should no longer be used for the routine treatment of alopecia areata. Topical irritants (e.g. dithranol, UVB and phenol) have also been recommended but are of limited value. PUVA treatment using high doses of UVA, may act via an immunosuppressive mechanism. The regrowth induced in most patients by these manoeuvres is temporary, patchy and cosmetically unsatisfactory.

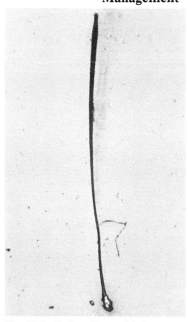

Fig. 20.3 Exclamation-mark hair.

TRICHOTILLOMANIA (see Ch. 16)

TRACTION ALOPECIA

Tight hair rollers, pony-tails, hot comb straighteners and other hair dressing procedures may all induce alopecia, usually at the borders of the scalp. The treatment is obvious, once the condition is recognised.

SCARRING (CICATRICIAL) ALOPECIA

Clinical features   Alopecia due to destruction of hair follicles has many causes (Table 20.1). The hair loss is irreversible.

Table 20.1 Causes of scarring alopecia

Physical injury
Fungal infection
Bacterial infection
Folliculitus decalvans
Neoplasm
Lichen planus
Chronic discoid lupus erythematosus
Scleroderma
Lichen sclerosus
Necrobiosis lipoidica
Sarcoidosis
Cicactricial pemphigoid
Pseudopelade

Management   Management entails identifying and halting the underlying disease. The scalp should be inspected for pustulation, follicular plugging or perifollicular scaling which may point to the aetiology (Figs. 20.4 and 20.5). If a fungal infection, e.g. Favus (*Trichophyton schoenleini*) is suspected, the scalp should be examined for fluorescence under ultra-violet light (Wood's light) and hairs removed for microscopy and culture.

If a biopsy is indicated, it should be taken from an early inflammatory lesion. Serial sections of follicles must be examined. Immunofluorescence studies may help.

If due to chronic discoid lupus erythematosus, scarring alopecia may be improved by wearing a sunhat, the use of sunscreens and potent topical steroids (clobetasol propionate ointment twice daily) or antimalarials (chloroquine sulphate 200 mg twice daily). Chloroquine may cause irreversible retinopathy so patients must be seen regularly by an ophthalmologist. Mepacrine 50–100 mg per day is preferred if available.

Systemic or intralesional steroids are occasionally indicated for scarring alopecia due to lichen planus.

Pustular disorders, e.g. folliculitis decalvans may require high doses of systemic antibiotics, such as flucloxacillin.

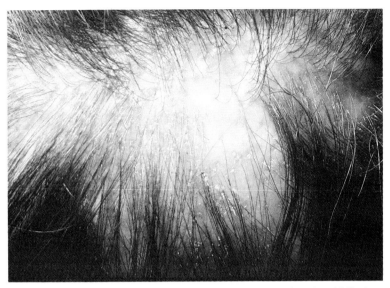

Fig. 20.4 Discoid lupus erythematosus may present with scarring alopecia and follicular plugging.

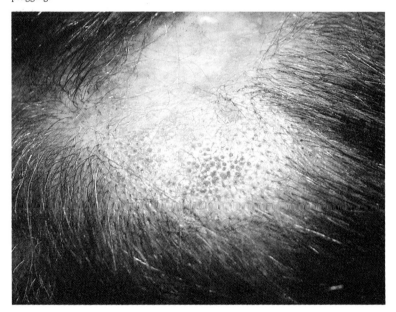

Fig. 20.5 Lichen planopilaris. Erythema, peri-follicular scaling and horny follicular plugging are obvious, surrounding an older white, smooth scarred area.

INFECTIONS AND INFESTATIONS (see Chs. 1 and 2)

NAIL

The structure of the nail is illustrated in Figure 20.6. The nail plate is formed from the nail matrix, a differentiated continuation of the dorsal

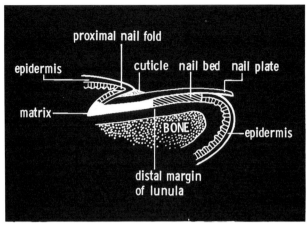

Fig. 20.6 The structure of the normal nail.

epidermis, and lies below the proximal nail fold. In health, the fingernails grow at about 1 cm per 3 months. The toe nails grow more slowly, approximately 1 cm per 6 months. These facts determine how long a treated nail dystrophy will take to return to normal.

General investigation and Management

The nail should be examined for changes in colour, shape or quality. The nail fold should also be inspected. The capilliaries may be seen more easily with a hand lens or in more detail by putting a drop of oil on the nail fold and using an ophthalmoscope set at +20.

A nail biopsy may be necessary (Fig. 20.7). A complete digital block is inserted using 2% lignocaine without adrenaline.

A local tumour of the nail bed or matrix can be sampled or excised using punch biopsy. A 2–3 mm punch is passed through the nail plate

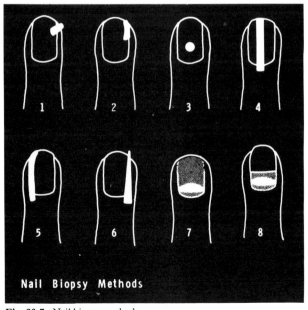

Fig. 20.7 Nail biopsy methods.

into the nail bed or matrix. A thick plate may need prior soaking in water to soften it.

An elliptical biopsy of the nail bed may be needed to investigate some tumours. The nail plate is separated from the nail bed and cut away to expose the lesion. A narrow longitudinal wedge of tissue is excised.

A matrix biopsy may be taken after removing the nail plate. The proximal matrix can be exposed by making incisions in the corners of the proximal nail fold and reflecting the fold.

For complete investigation of nail dystrophies, a well-orientated specimen containing nail matrix, bed and plate is required. Two parallel incisions are made, carried down to bone and extended from the proximal nail fold to the tip of the finger. The width between these incisions should not exceed 2 mm or the nail may remain split. A rectangular specimen is gently dissected off the bone using sharp, curved scissors. The more lateral the biopsy, the better the cosmetic result.

Nail biopsies are contra-indicated in patients with diabetes, scleroderma or peripheral vascular disease.

NAIL INFECTIONS

Acute paronychia

Clinical features   This bacterial infection of the nail fold is frequent in nail biters with a damaged cuticle. There is redness, swelling, tenderness and pain around the nail fold. The commonest causative organism is *Staphylococcus aureus*

Management   Most require incision and drainage as well as systemic antibiotics, e.g. flucloxacillin 250 mg four times a day.

Herpetic whitlow

Clinical features   *Herpes simplex* infection, an occupational hazard particularly of nurses and oral specialists, may simulate an acute bacterial paronychia. It is extremely painful. In the early stages it may be possible to see grouped vesicles. A Tzank preparation will demonstrate giant cells and the virus can be cultured from vesicle fluid.

Management   The infection is self-limiting but it may take 3 weeks for the lesions to dry up entirely. Topical 5% idoxuridine in dimethyl sulphoxide may be applied 3-hourly in the vesicular stage. A 5% acyclovir cream is also effective. Pus is not formed so incision is unhelpful.

Chronic paronychia

Clinical features   This is common in patients with hands endlessly immersed in water. The cuticle is damaged and *Candida albicans* and various bacteria invade

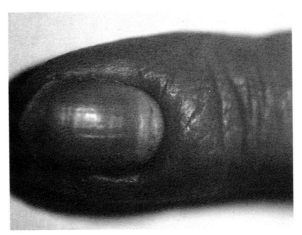

Fig. 20.8 Chronic paronychia with a swollen proximal nail fold and loss of the cuticle.

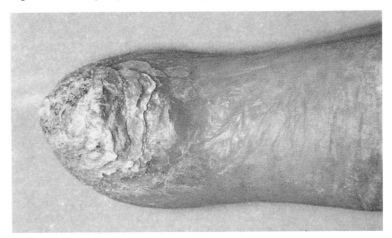

Fig. 20.9 Nail plate infection by *Candida albicans*. This can be difficult to distinguish clinically from tinea unguium.

the hydrated nail fold causing erythema and swelling (Fig. 20.8). Nail plate irregularities develop due to matrix inflation. *Candida albicans* may infect the nail plate and be difficult to distinguish from a dermatophyte infection (Fig. 20.9). *Pseudomonas aeruginosa* often invades the abnormal nail bed producing a greenish discolouration. There may be intermittent acute episodes if more virulent organisms invade.

Management
The finger must be kept dry. Prolonged occlusion with rubber gloves will only increase maceration so they should be worn for short periods and lined with cotton. An imidazole cream massaged into the nail fold twice daily for 6–12 weeks will eventually eradicate *Candida albicans* but the nail must be treated until a normal cuticle is formed. 3% thymol in chloroform or 15% sulphacetamide in 50% alcohol applied to the nail folds three or four times a day will inhibit *Candida albicans* and *Pseudomonas aeruginosa*, eliminating unsightly discolouration. Ketoconazole 200 mg/day may be very effective treatment if the nail plate

is infected. However, although oral ketoconazole is well tolerated by the majority of patients, there is an attendant risk of impaired liver function, which has been detected in 0.1–0.3% of those treated—5 deaths from liver disease have been recorded. Evidently the benefits of treatment must be carefully weighed against possible hepatic toxicity. In particularly resistant cases, surgical removal of the abnormal nail fold may be necessary.

Tinea unguium

Clinical features   *Trichophyton rubrum, Trichophyton interdigitale* and *Epidermophyton floccosum* may all infect the nails but there is usually a focus elsewhere, e.g. in the toe webs. The great toe nails are most commonly involved. The nail becomes thickened with onycholysis and subungual hyperkeratosis. The diagnosis should be confirmed by seeing hyphae in scrapings or culturing fungus. Unfortunately, in up to 10% of cases, culture may be negative. Scrapings can also be sent for routine histology to identify fungus using a PAS stain. Fungus may invade a nail abnormal for some other reason, e.g. trauma. If the fungus is eliminated, the nail abnormality may persist and the risk of re-infection is high.

Psoriasis of the nails may simulate a fungal infection (see below).

Management   Management is difficult, especially of the slowly-growing toe nails. Topical agents do not penetrate enough to destroy the fungus. Systemic antifungal agents (griseofulvin 500–1500 mg/day; ketoconazole 200 mg/day but see above warning) must be taken daily until the nail is completely normal, up to 2 years for toe nails. Compliance is often poor and recurrences common even after a successful 'cure', so it may be more sensible to recommend keeping the nail trimmed and to avoid systemic treatment.

ACQUIRED NAIL DYSTROPHIES

Ingrowing toe nails

Clinical features   Ingrowing toe nails, affecting the big toes, are common in young adults. The primary abnormality in the majority is a large lateral nail fold. Ill-fitting shoes (Fig. 20.10), hyperhydrosis or incorrect cutting contribute to the problem. A small proportion have congenital malalignment of the nail plate (Fig. 20.11)

The nail fold becomes erythematous and swollen and in the later stages there may be exuberant granulation tissue. A spicule of nail may grow into the nail fold, perpetuating the problem.

Management   Management should initially aim to reduce the acute inflammation and treat secondary infection. Potassium permanganate (1-10 000) soaks and

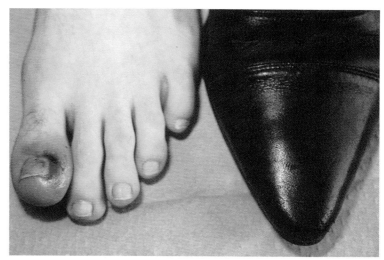

Fig. 20.10 Ingrowing toe-nail caused by a combination of large lateral nail folds and narrow shoes.

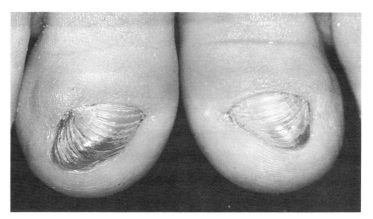

Fig. 20.11 Congenital malalignment of the nail plate may predispose to ingrowing toe-nails.

local antibiotic creams may be helpful. Exuberant granulation tissue can be inhibited by silver nitrate, gentle cautery or cryotherapy. Spicules of nail should be removed. Some patients need the entire nail removed, and as the new nail forms small cottonwool pledgets should be inserted under the corners to prevent recurrence. The nail should be cut straight across and wide-fitting shoes or sandals worn. More radical surgical procedures may be required such as wedge resection of the nail fold and nail bed or even total ablation of the nail bed.

Congenital malalignment of the nail plate should be considered. This abnormality can be corrected surgically if diagnosis and correction of the defect is undertaken by 2 years of age. If not recognised many patients will present at an older age with onychogryphosis or other abnormalities.

Brittle nails

Clinical features   Repeated immersion of the hands in water and detergents, followed by drying, causes distal separation of the nail plate into layers, distal onychoschizia. Brittle nails may also be a sign of peripheral vascular insufficiency, anaemia or hypothyroidism.

Management   The treatment is that of the underlying condition.

Onycholysis

Clinical features   Patchy distal separation of the nail plate from the nail bed may be due to frequent immersion in water. Onycholysis is also caused by psoriasis (Fig. 20.12), fungal infections or photosensitizers (tetracyclines, porphyrins).

Pseudomonas infection beneath the loosened nail causes blue black discolouration.

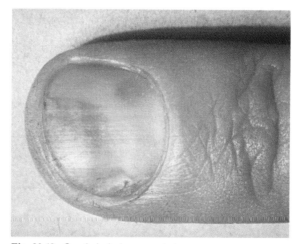

Fig. 20.12   Onycholysis due to psoriasis.

Management   The nail should be trimmed. A 15% solution of sulphacetamide in 50% alcohol or 3% thymol in chloroform applied daily to the nail bed inhibits infection and may encourage reattachment.

TUMOURS OF NAIL APPARATUS

Digital mucus cyst

Clinical features   This cystic lesion occurs most commonly on the distal phalanx near the base of the nail (Fig. 20.13). It may depress the nail matrix and cause a furrow in the nail plate. The cyst often connects directly with the joint space.

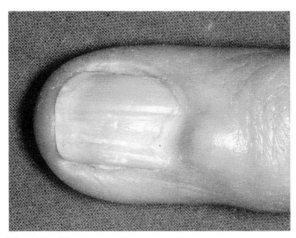

Fig. 20.13   Digital mucous cyst.

Management   Management is difficult. Repeated pricking and draining of the cysts have been recommended; however, there is a risk of introducing infection. Cryotherapy has been recommended but may cause permanent nail matrix damage. Cysts may be removed surgically but the dissection must be carried down to the joint space. There is a risk of recurrence with all these forms of treatment.

Glomus tumours

These painful, bluish subungual nodules require excision.

Pigmented lesions

Clinical features   Longitudinal brown bands in the nail folds are common in coloured races and are benign (Fig. 20.14). In Caucasians an acquired brown-black line is a worrying sign, especially if the proximal nail fold is involved.

Early biopsy must be performed to exclude malignant melanoma. Malignant melanoma may also present as an amelanoic growth in the nail bed so any unusual lesion should be removed for histological examination.

NAILS IN SKIN DISEASE

Eczema

Irregular transverse ridging and less commonly coarse pitting are seen in both endogenous eczema and exogenous (contact irritant) eczema when it affects the terminal phalanges. The nail changes usually improve as the eczema is treated but endogenous changes may persist.

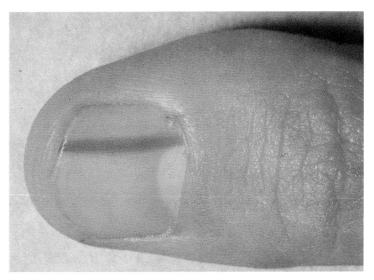

Fig. 20.14 Benign lentigo in a caucasian. An acquired pigmented line may be due to malignant melanoma especially if the proximal nail fold is involved.

Psoriasis

Pitting (Fig. 20.15), onycholysis and thickening usually affect the majority of the nails symmetrically. Pustular psoriasis may cause complete loss of the nail. Psoriatic nail dystrophy fluctuates like psoriasis elsewhere.

Management Unfortunately, topical treatments are unhelpful. Steroids may be injected into the nail matrix and produce temporary improvement but relapse is common and local atrophy a worrying complication. High intensity PUVA has also been used locally and may produce remission. Etretinate 25–75 mg/day, is not useful for the common psoriatic nail dystrophy but acropustular psoriasis may be benefited.

Lichen planus

Clinical features Longitudinal ridging and fragility are the mildest changes of lichen planus and may reverse spontaneously. Unfortunately, irreversible disease may also occur. The cuticle hypertrophies, adheres to the nail plate and grows forward forming a triangular 'scar' (pterygium) (Fig. 20.16), eventually completely destroying the nail. Sometimes the nails undergo progressive total atrophy without pterygium formation. The diagnosis of lichen planus should be confirmed by longitudinal biopsy if there is any doubt.

Management Treatment with systemic steroids (prednisolone 40 mg/day) for some weeks may halt the progression of destructive disease but there is a risk of

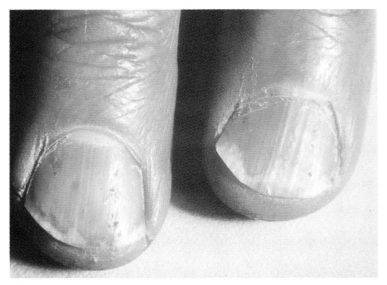

Fig. 20.15 Small 'thimble' pitting in psoriasis.

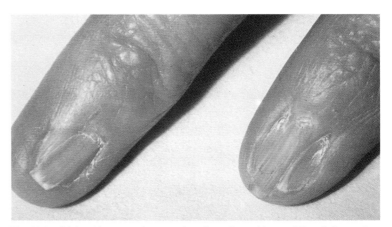

Fig. 20.16 Lichen planus causing pterygium formation and irreversible nail destruction.

relapse when treatment is withdrawn. A powerful steroid (clobetasol propionate ointment) applied locally with occlusion may occasionally prove useful.

FURTHER READING

Baran R, Dawber R P R (eds) 1984 Diseases of the nails and their management. Blackwell Scientific Publications, London

Orfanos C E, Montagna W, Stuttgen G (eds) 1981 Hair research: status and future aspects. Springer-Verlag, Berlin

Rentoul J R, Young R E, Beastall G, Wallace M, Morley P 1983 The investigation of hirsutism. British Journal of Dermatology 108: 224

Rook A, Dawber R (eds) 1982 Diseases of the hair and scalp. Blackwell Scientific Publications, London

Sammon P D (ed) 1978 The nails in disease. Heinemann London

21. Topical Therapy— a Review

The skin is the most accessible organ that doctors have to treat and therefore it is natural that, if possible, therapeutic agents should be applied to the skin rather than taken orally. The obvious advantage is that the highest concentration of the drug is at the site of the pathology and only small amounts are transported to distant sites so that systemic side-effects are kept to the minimum. As a general rule topical therapy is more effective for epidermal than dermal diseases; the former includes eczema, psoriasis, fungal infections and superficial bacterial infections such as impetigo.

VEHICLES FOR TOPICAL DRUGS

Lotions

These are used when the pathological state is acute, e.g. with 'weeping' of serum. Lotions may also be used in moist, intertriginous areas. The scalp is another area where lotions may be used because patients do not like greasy substances on the hair.

Lotions are probably the least effective of bases as they evaporate quickly and thus tend to have a relatively short duration of action. For a continuous therapeutic effect, lotions would have to be applied every 2 or 3 hours. Lotions tend to be pleasant to use and have a high degree of patient compliance.

Creams

These have a high water content with a smaller proportion of oils or fats than ointments and are essentially emulsions. Creams should be used for subacute conditions in which there may be some crusting, and they may be used in intertriginous areas. As creams have a high water content they last for a relatively short duration on the skin due to evaporation of water. However, because of this they will cool the skin and have an 'anti-irritation' effect. To maintain the continuous effect of a drug in a cream base it should be applied every 4 hours. Creams are pleasant to use as they 'rub in' and there is a high degree of patient compliance.

Creams should not be used on dry, scaly, cracked skin, as the cooling effect may well aggravate the epidermal changes.

Ointments

These are 'greasy'. They consist mainly or totally of oils or similar substances. Although some may mix with water, as a general rule they should not be used for the moist intertriginous areas. Ointments are more effective than creams or lotions as they are more persistent and thus act as a depot for the drug. In addition, they form an artificial barrier, decreasing water loss from the skin which in turn increases absorption of the drug due to the increase in local humidity. Ointments tend to last on the skin for 6−8 hours and thus only need to be applied three times a day for continuous treatment of the skin lesions.

Pastes

These are ointments to which zinc oxide has been added to stiffen them. Pastes are used to stop spread of the drug to the surrounding skin. They are only applied once or twice daily especially if the drug in question is a potential irritant, e.g. dithranol.

QUANTITY OF TOPICAL PREPARATION

It is important that the appropriate quantity of topical preparation is prescribed, otherwise the patient will receive ineffective therapy. Unlike the prescribing of tablets, when a precise number is dispensed for a specific time, patients with rashes are arbitrarily given tubes of creams and ointments of varying sizes. A simple working rule is that it takes approximately 30 g of cream or ointment to cover all the skin of an average adult. Thus, if the approximate surface area of the skin disease can be ascertained it is possible to estimate the quantity of ointment needed for one application and then multiply this figure by the frequency of application and duration of use before the next appointment. The 'rule of nines' for working out the extent of skin involved is a useful guide. In general, patients with extensive skin lesions are often given insufficient quantities of topical preparations, leading to insufficient drug to clear the eruption.

TOPICAL STEROIDS

These are the most widely prescribed drugs in dermatology and have revolutionized the therapy of inflammatory skin disorders. Although

recently topical steroids have had a bad 'press', this is not justified.
Topical steroids may have side-effects but if they are used correctly, the
side-effects are mostly avoidable. It is important to realise that there is
now a considerable range in the potency of topical steroids and obviously
side effects depend on the potency and the duration of use. Using very
potent topical steroids for a short period is relatively safe. Two other
factors will influence side-effects from topical steroids and these are skin
thickness and hydration. If the skin is thin as on the face or moist as in
the intertriginous areas, there will be increased risk of skin damage.

The side effects seen with topical steroids are due to the fact that
steroids will cause breakdown of collagen and inhibit fibroblasts from
forming new collagen. This, coupled with epidermal atrophy and
flattening of the dermo/epidermal interface, results in steroid (shear)
purpura, telangiectasia (Figs. 21.1 and 21.2) due to increased
transparency and in the development of striae (Fig. 21.3).

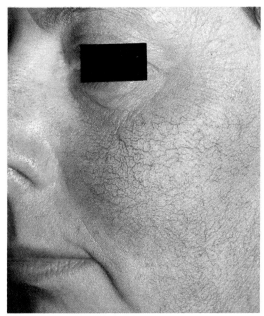

Fig. 21.1 Telangiectasia on the cheek from prolonged use of a strong topical steroid.

Topical steroids will also suppress the body's reaction to local infection
and therefore should be avoided if infection is suspected. If these are used
in error they will alter the clinical presentation of the infection and make
the diagnosis that much more difficult, e.g. tinea incognita.

An unusual side-effect of topical steroid therapy is sometimes seen
when potent topical steroids have been used on the face for treating
seborrhoeic eczema. Although initially helpful, eventually they lose their
beneficial effect and the eruption begins to break through. If the potent
topical steroid is stopped abruptly there is often a rebound with
worsening of the condition with the development of papules and
pustules. Classically, this condition is seen around the mouth and has

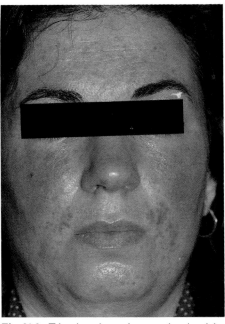

Fig. 21.2 Telangiectasia, erythema, and peri-oral dermatitis after long term (inappropriate) treatment of seborrhoeic eczema with potent topical steroids.

been termed circumoral dermatitis (Figs. 21.2 and 21.4). Treatment consists of weaning the patient off the potent topical steroid by gradual reductions in the potency over a period of 3 months. Oral tetracycline is often beneficial and many recommend its routine use.

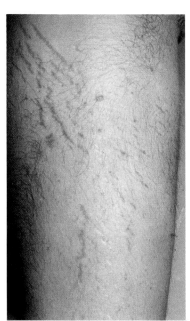

Fig. 21.3 Striae on the inner thigh from potent topical steroids.

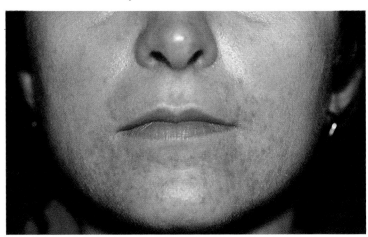

Fig. 21.4 Peri-oral dermatitis.

Systemic side-effects from absorption of topical steroids are far more a theoretical than a practical hazard. Unnecessarily large quantities of high-potency steroids are required to produce suppression of the pituitary-adrenal axis. Cushingoid features are seen only after long-term treatment with high-potency steroids in large quantities. This situation is largely avoidable by using other treatment regimens.

In the past it has not been appreciated that topical steroids have a wide range of potency. The therapeutic effect and unfortunately risk of side-effects are directly proportional to the steroid potency and duration of treatment. This risk/benefit ratio should always be considered. It has been proved helpful to classify topical steroids into weak, moderate, potent and very potent. This classification is based on a vasoconstrictor assay. The practising physician should learn to use one steroid from each of the four groups and not vary his prescribing. In this way the risks of side-effects will be decreased.

As a general rule, potent and very potent topical steroids should not be used on the face and intertriginous areas. It should be stressed that a short course of a potent topical steroid may do the patient more good than long-term use of a weak- or moderate-potency steroid, which only partially suppresses the pathology.

TOPICAL ANTIBIOTICS

There is a high incidence of sensitivity to topical antibiotics, particularly in diseased skin. Widespread and prolonged use is discouraged by many bacteriologists because of the risks of drug resistance. It is now considered more appropriate to use short courses of systemic antibiotics for skin infections such as impetigo, although non-antibiotic antibacterials are acceptable. In the case of mixed infections such as in venous ulcers, antiseptics with a low sensitizing potential, such as eusol or gentian violet, should be used.

There are relatively few indications for using topical antibiotics in conjunction with topical steroids, although the combination of steroid with chinoform is often useful in secondarily-infected eczema combined with a course of systemic antibiotics.

One of the indications for topical antibiotics is to eradicate staphylococci from carrier sites such as the anterior nares, axillae or groins. Sodium fusidate is probably the best preparation as the incidence of sensitization is very low.

A new topical antibiotic, 2% mupirocin, has great potential for the treatment of primary bacterial skin infections. So far staphylococci have not shown resistance.

TOPICAL ANTIHISTAMINES AND LOCAL ANAESTHETICS

These preparations have little or no part to play in the treatment of skin diseases. Both groups of drugs are potent sensitizers. Although they may relieve irritation, it is far better to suppress the primary skin disease with appropriate treatment.

GENTIAN VIOLET AND MAGENTA PAINTS

These preparations have been used for many years in dermatology. They have anti-inflammatory, antibacterial, antifungal and astringent effects.

The indications for using these preparations have decreased with the advent of more specific antimicrobial and antifungal drugs, but they are still useful in a number of conditions. Magenta paint is spirit-based and therefore will sting when applied to an eroded area or fissure. Gentian violet is usually applied in aqueous solution. The indications for magenta paint are for intertriginous eczema and mixed infections in these areas. Aqueous gentian violet is useful for weeping erosions, as may occur in bullous disorders and for treating venous ulcers. Patient compliance is variable because of possible staining of clothing.

POTASSIUM PERMANGANATE SOAKS

A lukewarm solution of potassium permanganate at a dilution of 1:8000 is helpful in acute weeping and blistering conditions, particularly on the palms and soles as may occur in acute eczema or fungal infections. The affected part should be immersed for 15 minutes approximately four times a day. In addition to its astringent properties, potassium permanganate is antibacterial and may stop secondary bacterial infection. Patients should be warned that potassium permanganate will stain the nails and skin.

ALUMINIUM ACETATE

This has long been in use as an astringent and as a treatment for hyperhidrosis. Burow's Solution contains about 13% of aluminium acetate and a 1:20 dilution of this is commonly used as a wet dressing.

SILVER NITRATE

Silver nitrate 0.5% in aqueous solution is an extremely valuable lotion with astringent and disinfectant properties. It is used as a wet dressing in infected eczema, gravitational ulcer and any other weeping or infected skin lesion. A 40% solution in alcohol has been used in the management of severe folliculitis. It has the disadvantage of staining the skin black but this is outweighed by rapid resolution of weeping and the control of superficial infection.

CAMPHOR

Camphor is added to shake lotions for its cooling and antipruritic effect, particularly in urticaria and lichen planus. It is also used in many chilblain preparations for the same reasons.

MENTHOL

Menthol is used similarly to camphor and the two are often combined in the one preparation. Both drugs probably act by inducing a feeling of cold which competitively inhibits itching.

ICHTHAMMOL (Ichthyol)

This has been used in dermatology for many generations. It is prepared by the destructive distillation of a bituminous shale with ammonium sulphate to form a sulphur rich substance. It is generally formulated in bases containing glycerin.

It is believed to have anti-inflammatory and vasoactive properties and has been used in the management of eczema, especially seborrhoeic and in rosacea. Its safety, patient acceptance and the symptomatic relief it gives are more than adequate reasons for its continuing popularity, despite the lack of evidence about its pharmacological activity.

SALICYLIC ACID

Salicylic acid is a keratolytic and it produces slow and painless destruction of the keratin. Its action on hyperplastic keratin is probably twofold: to decrease keratinocyte adhesion and to increase water-binding, thus hydrating the keratin. It can be used in concentrations of 0.5–60% in a collodion, gel, cream or ointment base or as an alcoholic solution.

Sensitization is unknown and irritation uncommon if care is taken to introduce low concentrations at first.

It enhances the percutaneous absorption of other agents and has been added to some topical corticosteroid preparations for this purpose.

SULPHUR

Sulphur is still used extensively in seborrhoeic conditions and in scabies as a 10% ointment. Its use in acne vulgaris is controversial as it may be comedogenic in animals. In seborrhoeic conditions it is often combined with many other agents so it is difficult to assess whether or not it has any specific activity. Sensitization is rare.

Sodium thiosulphate 20% solution is used in the management of widespread tinea versicolor but it is being displaced by the imidazole antifungals.

TAR

Coal tar, a thick black viscous fluid, is a product of distillation of coal in the production of gas. The chief constituents are benzene, naphthalene, and phenols with small quantities of pyridine and quinoline. There are variations in its composition.

It is an antipruritic and keratoplastic. It is used in eczema, psoriasis and other conditions. Patient compliance is often a problem but it produces gratifying results in chronic eczema, particularly atopic.

Coal tar is usually prescribed in ointment or paste bases and tar impregnated bandages, useful in the management of childhood atopic eczema, are available. It is also available as a solution in alcohol which is useful for preparation of lotion forms or for adding to baths.

It may cause irritation and acne-like eruptions of the skin. It also has a photosensitizing action. Tar is carcinogenic in experimental animals. However, there are few reports of carcinomata developing as a result of therapy, despite its widespread and prolonged use.

DITHRANOL (Anthralin)

Dithranol is a synthetic derivative of chrysarobin and it is used widely in a variety of bases including pastes, ointments, paints and waxsticks. There are also special formulations for the scalp. It is used in the treatment of psoriasis; treatment is commonly started with a paste or ointment containing 0.1%, the strength being increased gradually. The face, skin flexures and genitalia are particularly sensitive and a strength of 0.01% initially applied three times a week has been suggested.

It stains normal skin dark brown or black and it is also irritating. For these reasons, it is usual to apply it in a base such as a paste that does not spread from the area of application. However, dithranol in soft paraffin is used in short contact therapy, i.e. applied for 30 minutes to 2 hours. It is often used in conjunction with salicyclic acid.

Julian L. Verbov

22. Systemic Therapy— a Review

Systemic therapy has an important place in dermatology and, of course, is often employed in combination with topical treatment.

Treatment of severe systemic disease may include corticosteroids, cytotoxic drugs, antimalarials and sometimes plasmapheresis in lupus erythematosus, oral d-penicillamine in systemic sclerosis and systemic corticosteroids in dermatomyositis. However, many cases of systemic lupus erythematosus may not require aggressive treatment.

ANTI-ANDROGENS

Cyproterone, an anti-androgen with the oestrogen ethinyloestradiol, is occasionally given to women with severe acne refractory to prolonged oral antibacterial therapy. It must be continued for at least 3 months before improvement is seen; such improvement probably occurs because it decreases sebum secretion, which is under androgen control.

Cyproterone is available in a tablet containing 2 mg cyproterone with 0.05 mg ethinyloestradiol. It is contraceptive, one tablet daily is taken for 21 days in monthly cycles starting on the 5th day of the menstrual cycle and then repeated after a 7-day interval, usually for several months. It is also of some use against mild to moderate hirsutism.

ANTIBIOTICS

Tetracyclines play an essential role in acne treatment. The usual dosage of oxytetracycline, the tetracycline of first choice, is 250 mg three times daily for 3–4 weeks, then 250 mg twice daily until improvement occurs. It should be taken before meals for maximum absorption and not with milk. Acceptable improvement may take many months and the duration of continuous treatment may vary from 3 months to 2 years. Other tetracyclines, and erythromycin or co-trimoxazole are recognised alternatives.

Patients with rosacea who do not respond to oxytetracycline 250 mg twice daily, which may be needed for up to 6 months, may be helped by oral metronidazole 200 mg three times a day for 3 weeks. The eye symptoms of rosacea also respond to systemic treatment.

Widespread impetigo, which is usually due to *Staphylococcus aureus* but may be complicated by streptococci, should be treated with a systemic antibiotic such as penicillin V, 250 mg four times a day for 10 days, or erythromycin, 250 mg four times a day for 10 days.

Treatment of staphlyococcal scalded skin syndrome (SSSS), which is due to a penicillin-resistant staphylococcus, is with systemic flucloxacillin, 250 mg four times daily; doses may be doubled in severe infections or sodium fusidate, 500 mg by mouth every 8 hours.

Streptococcal erysipelas merits intramuscular crystalline penicillin for 24 hours followed by oral penicillin V. Widespread or recurrent boils need systemic antibiotics but the possibility of nasal carriage of staphylococci must be considered.

A systemic antibiotic is often needed for cellulitis complicating stasis ulceration. Cellulitis should be remembered as one of the causes of pain associated with a gravitational ulcer (see Ch. 6).

ANTIFUNGAL DRUGS

Griseofulvin is indicated for ringworm, particularly if spreading and not controlled by topical agents. The usual adult dosage is 500 mg daily with breakfast. Tinea cruris and tinea capitis need 6 weeks treatment but nail infection (tinea unguium) must be treated for between 18 months and 2 years.

Ketoconazole is indicated in griseofulvin-unresponsive ringworm and in severe candidal infections. Given as 200 mg daily for 3 weeks only, it also treats the Pityrosporum organism causing pityriasis versicolor in cases unresponsive to topical treatment. (There have been reports of liver damage and interference with steroid hormone synthesis with ketoconazole. See Ch. 20.)

ANTIVIRAL DRUGS

Severe widespread and painful herpes simplex, particularly in patients with altered cellular immunity, such as children with atopic eczema, is an indication for intravenous or oral acycloguanosine (acyclovir). This antiviral agent inhibits herpes virus replication but does not interfere with production of host DNA.

Acyclovir has a place in the therapy of herpes zoster in immunocompromised patients and may reduce post-herpetic neuralgia in the elderly.

Zoster immune globulin may be useful in patients with herpes zoster.

ANTIHISTAMINES

Antihistamines, such as hydroxyzine, promethazine and trimeprazine are useful in the itching of eczema but the more recently introduced, non-sedative ones are not effective in eczema (see Ch. 7). Suggested doses are:
1. Hydroxyzine—25 mg three or four times daily
2. Promethazine—25 mg at night, increased if necessary to
        50–75 mg at night
3. Trimeprazine—10 mg three or four times daily.

Unfortunately, there is no specific anti-itch preparation for eczema. These drugs also help the troublesome irritation in lichen planus.

Many well-tried antihistamines are available for the treatment of urticaria and angio-oedema but the new non-sedative antihistamines, terfenadine and astemizole, are especially useful. The doses are:
1. Astemizole—10 mg daily
2. Terfenadine—60 mg twice daily.

Oral antihistamines are usually adequate but acute urticaria may need an intravenous antihistamine such as chlorpheniramine (10–20 mg); intramuscular or subcataneous adrenaline 1:1000 (0.5 ml) or intravenous hydrocortisone sodium succinate (100 mg).

ANTIMETABOLITES

Severe psoriasis not responding to topical therapy may be treated with antimetabolites such as methotrexate or azathioprine.

The dose range for methotrexate is from 10–25 mg once a week by intravenous, intramuscular or oral routes adjusted according to the patient's response. For azathioprine the dose is 100 mg daily, increased after 2 weeks to 200 mg (exceptionally to 300 mg daily). This is continued as required and reduced when remission is obtained. The haematological parameters must be monitored regularly.

Lymphoma is often treated by systemic anti-metabolites, often in combination, or by PUVA.

PUVA is the combination of psoralens orally (8-methoxypsoralen) and long-wave ultra-violet light (UVA). It is used in severe widespread psoriasis unresponsive to topical applications. The eyes must be protected with special spectacles during, and for 24 hours after, PUVA treatment (see Ch. 9).

CORTICOSTEROIDS

Systemic corticosteroids, ACTH or long-acting tetracosactrin 2 mg weekly may be needed in acute severe eczema and a small maintenance dose indicated in severe chronic eczema. However, only a short course of systemic steroids or ACTH should be the aim. Prednisolone 20–30 mg daily is suggested and the dose reduced gradually over 4–6 weeks.

ACTH, 80 units weekly or tetracosactrin can be given and this should also be reduced gradually.

Occasionally in extensive irritant lichen planus a 3-week course of systemic corticosteroids is indicated; it starts with 30 mg prednisolone daily, reducing to nil over the 3 weeks.

The most severe form of erythema multiforme, Stevens-Johnson syndrome, may require systemic corticosteroids. Minor erythema multiforme may be relieved by oral antihistamine therapy. Chlortetracycline mouthwash (see Formulary), to each 15 ml of which is added triamcinolone 2 mg, often helps the mouth ulcer. 15 ml should be used three times a day.

Erythroderma is a complication of psoriasis, eczema, drug reaction, pre-reticulosis, or can be of unknown cause. Topical and systemic steroids (up to 60 mg prednisolone a day) are often required until the condition is controlled.

Systemic corticosteroids, ACTH or short-acting tetracosactrin, and immunosuppressants, particularly azathioprine, are indicated in bullous pemphigoid and pemphigus vulgaris. Large doses may be required. Such patients should be hospitalized.

In the middle-aged healthy patient with herpes zoster, systemic steroid therapy started early reduces the likelihood of post-herpetic neuralgia. Prednisolone 60 mg daily is given for 1 week, then 30 mg daily for 1 week, then 15 mg daily for a final week. This regimen may eventually be replaced by the wider use of acyclovir.

Recovery from impaired adrenocortical function caused by prolonged systemic therapy is slow. Patients should be given a steroid warning card and should carry it for at least 6 months after cessation of systemic steroid therapy. They should also have a supply of oral steroid to use in emergencies such as trauma, surgery or infection. Corticosteroids may worsen diabetes.

In patients with dyspeptic side-effects, enteric-coated prednisolone or soluble betamethasone may be helpful.

RETINOIDS

In most countries, retinoids are available for hospital use only. For their use in children see Ch. 13. Etretinate is used to treat severe intractable plaque psoriasis and peripheral pustular psoriasis, often with spectacularly good results. It has a marked effect on keratinising epithelia. The clinical effect starts after 2−3 weeks of therapy, reaching maximum benefit after 4−6 weeks.

Etretinate dosage is 0.75−1 mg/kg bodyweight daily in divided doses for 2−4 weeks. If no response is seen within 4 weeks and in the absence of toxicity, this dose may be increased in steps of 10 mg weekly to a maximum daily dose of 1.5 mg/kg. When a response has been obtained the dosage should be reduced to 0.5 mg/kg daily and taken for a further 6−8 weeks.

Most patients suffer from dry, cracked lips when an adequate dose is given. Other side-effects include mild transient alopecia, generalized pruritus and epistaxis. Etretinate is teratogenic and must be avoided in women who may become pregnant, unless contraceptive measures are taken during treatment and for 1 year after a course of the drug.

Another oral retinoid isotretinoin (13-cis retinoic acid) is indicated in some patients with severe cystic acne often with very gratifying results. Again, women of child-bearing age given isotretinoin must practise effective contraception for 1 month before treatment and for at least 1 month afterwards as it is teratogenic, although its half-life is not as long as etretinate.

The initial dosage for isotretinoin is 0.5 mg/kg bodyweight daily for 4 weeks. Subsequent dosage will depend on response:

1. Early improvement: continue with initial dosage for a further 8–12 weeks
2. Little or no initial improvement but the drug well tolerated. 1 mg/kg bodyweight for a further 8–12 weeks
3. Intolerance to the initial dosage: 0.1–0.2 mg/kg bodyweight daily for 8–12 weeks.

Doses up to 2 mg/kg/day may be required in patients with extensive disease.

EVENING PRIMROSE OIL

Oral evening primrose oil providing gamma-linolenic acid may improve the skin in atopic eczema. Adult dosage is four 500 mg capsules twice a day; for children, four 250 mg capsules twice a day.

SODIUM CROMOGLYCATE AND DIETARY MATTERS

If food allergy appears to worsen atopic eczema, oral sodium cromoglycate can be tried (25–50 mg daily four times a day, 30 minutes before meals) with short-term dietary exclusion of the appropriate foods (e.g. cow's milk, eggs). Medical or dietetic supervision is essential. Soya protein substitutes are available for patients with milk intolerance but allergy to soya may also develop. Goat's milk is contraindicated as a substitute for cow's milk in infants. It has dangers such as a high solute load, deficiency of folic acid and probably vitamin B_{12}: it may also be deficient in vitamins C and D and there is a risk of bacterial infection.

Formulary

See also: Chapter 21   Topical therapy
            Chapter 22   Systemic therapy
            The index

ALUMINIUM CHLORIDE SOLUTION

A 6.2%–20% alcoholic solution is used for topical application as an astringent and antiperspirant. A 30% solution is used in athlete's foot (see also Burow's Solution).

BETAMETHASONE PHOSPHATE SOLUTION

This may be prepared by adding effervescent tablets of betamethasone phosphate (0.5 mg) to water. It is usually employed as a 0.5–1.0% solution.

BUROW'S SOLUTION (Aluminium Acetotartrate Solution)

This contains about 10.5% of aluminium acetotartrate.

CHLORHEXIDINE MOUTHWASH

Chlorhexidine gluconate solution	1 ml
Alcohol (95%)	7 ml
Freshly boiled and cooled water	to 100 ml

CHLORTETRACYCLINE MOUTHWASH

Chlortetracycline	2%
Glycerin	10%
Water	to 100 ml

15 ml is used as a mouthwash 3 times a day for the treatment of aphthous ulceration.

CULLEN AND CHILDERS SOLUTION

For scabies identification

Tetracycline	500 mg
Glycerin	20 ml
Absolute Alcohol	to 100 ml

HYDROGEN PEROXIDE SOLUTION

A 1.5% solution is used as a mouthwash in the treatment of acute stomatitis and as a deodorant gargle. A 3% solution is used for the cleansing of cutaneous ulcers.

IMIDAZOLE ANTIFUNGAL AGENTS

These include clotrimazole, econazole and miconazole. Clotrimazole and econazole are used as 1% creams and lotions. Miconazole is applied as a 2% cream or dusting powder.

LASSAR'S PASTE (see Zinc and Salicyclic Acid Paste)

LIGNOCAINE MOUTHWASH

This is prepared by diluting lignocaine hydrochloride viscous preparations to a final concentration of 0.5%.

METHOTREXATE

Methotrexate is given by mouth, intramuscularly and intravenously in the treatment of psoriasis. Single weekly doses of 10−25 mg may be given by mouth or injection. Alternatively, 2.5 mg may be given by mouth every 12 hours for 3 doses or every 8 hours for 4 doses each week or 2.5 mg may be given daily by mouth for 5 days out of 7.

It is essential that examination of blood and tests of renal and liver function should be made before, during and after each course of treatment with methotrexate. If there is a severe fall in the white cell or platelet counts, the drug should be withdrawn.

POTASSIUM IODIDE ORAL SOLUTION

Potassium Iodide	100 g
Water	to 100 ml

SILVER SULPHADIAZINE CREAM

A 1% cream is used for the prevention and treatment of infection, particularly by *Pseudomonas aeruginosa* in burns. The cream is usually applied daily to a thickness of 3–5 mm.

ST MARK'S LOTION

Phenol	1 g
Zinc oxide	2 g
Calamine	1 g
Glycerol	2 ml
Rose Water	3.5 ml
Mixture of Magnesium Hydroxide	to 28 ml

TINEA VERSICOLOR SHAMPOO

Sulphur	2%
Salicyclic Acid	2%

incorporated in a shampoo base such as a Soap Spirit or a sodium lauryl sulphate preparation.

TRIAMCINOLONE MOUTHWASH

Daily totals of 0.75 mg, 1.5 mg or 3 mg may be given in chlortetracycline mouthwash. Each application must be measured carefully.

CAMPHOR AND MENTHOL IN CALAMINE LOTION

Camphor	0.5%
Menthol	0.5%
Calamine Lotion	to 100 ml

SALICYLIC ACID AND SULPHUR OINTMENT

Salicylic Acid	2%
Sulphur	2%
Hydrous Ointment	to 100 g

ZINC AND SALICYLIC ACID PASTE (Lassar's Paste)

Zinc Oxide	24 g
Salicylic Acid	2 g
Starch	24 g
White Soft Paraffin	50 g

ZINC SULPHATE SOLUTION

Zinc Sulphate	220 mg
Glycerin	1 ml
Water	to 5 ml

5 ml to be taken twice daily.

The approximate clinical effectiveness of topical corticosteroids

Very potent	Clobetasol propionate	0.05%
	Diflucortolone valerate	0.3%
	Fluocinolone acetonide	0.2%
	Halcinonide	0.1%
Potent	Betamethasone dipropionate	0.05%
	Betamethasone valerate	0.1%
	Desoxymethasone	0.25%
	Difluocortolone valerate	0.1%
	Fluocinolone acetonide	0.025%
	Fluocinonide	0.05%
Moderate to mild	Clobetasone butyrate	0.05%
	Fluclorolone acetonide	0.025%
	Fluocortolone hexanoate	0.1%
	with fluocortolone pivalate	0.1%
	Flumethasone pivalate	0.02%
	Flurandrenolone	0.125%
	Hydrocortisone	1% with urea 10%
	Hydrocortisone butyrate	0.1%
	Triamcinolone acetonide	0.1%
Weak	Hydrocortisone	0.5%, 1%
	Methylprednisolone acetate	0.2%

Substances are given in alphabetical order and are of approximately similar clinical effectiveness within the four groups. However relatively few clinical comparisons have been published and there may be considerable variations in response between individuals.

Index